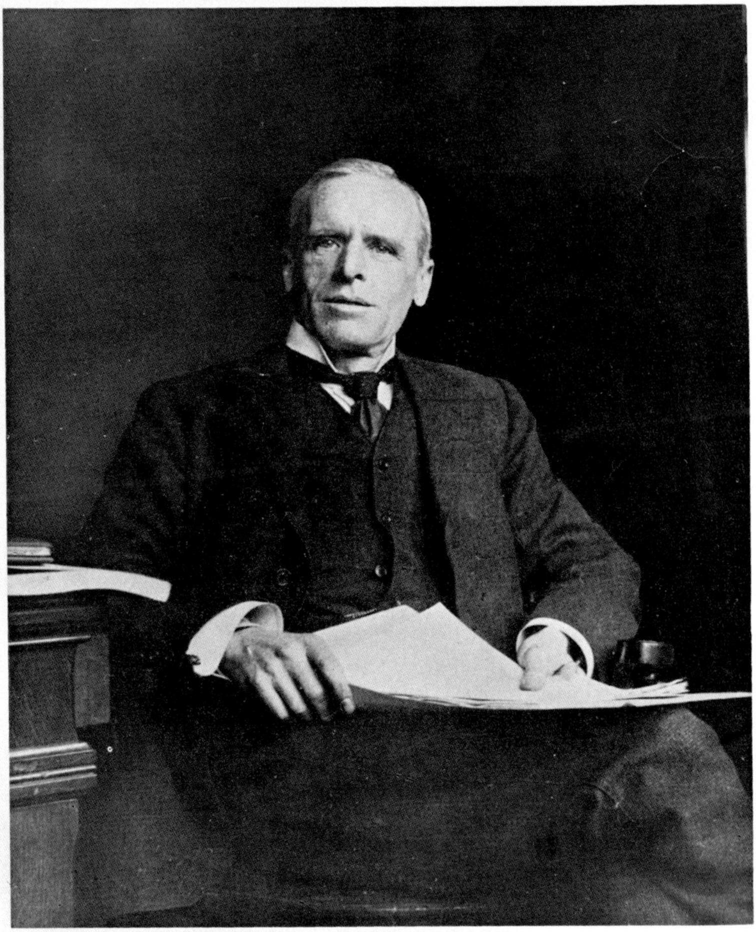

Ernest H. Starling, C.M.G., F.R.S.

Second Printing

A PRIMER OF VENOUS PRESSURE

BY

GEORGE E. BURCH, M.D., M.A.C.P.

Henderson Professor of Medicine, Tulane University School of Medicine; Physician-in-Chief, Tulane Medicine Unit, Charity Hospital of Louisiana; Consultant in Cardiovascular Diseases, Veterans Administration Hospital, Touro Infirmary, Ochsner Clinic, Ochsner Foundation Hospital; Consultant in Medicine, Southern Baptist Hospital, Hotel Dieu, Illinois Central Clinic, Mercy Hospital, U.S. Public Health Service Hospital, New Orleans, and East Jefferson Hospital

CHARLES C THOMAS · PUBLISHER

Springfield · Illinois · U.S.A.

Published and Distributed Throughout the World by

CHARLES C THOMAS • PUBLISHER

BANNERSTONE HOUSE

301-327 East Lawrence Avenue, Springfield, Illinois, U.S.A.

ISBN 0-398-02556-8

First Printing, 1950
Second Printing, 1972

With THOMAS BOOKS *careful attention is given to all details of manufacturing and design. It is the Publisher's desire to present books that are satisfactory as to their physical qualities and artistic possibilities and appropriate for their particular use.* THOMAS BOOKS *will be true to those laws of quality that assure a good name and good will.*

Printed in the United States of America
N-1

Dedicated to

VIVIAN GERARD BURCH

in appreciative recognition of her companionship and untiring assistance and encouragement in all of my endeavors.

PREFACE

Because interest in the veins, venous pressure and venous circulation has been increasing rapidly in recent years, this monograph is reissued. The growing interest is prompted by the new developments in cardiovascular surgery, cardiac catheterization and related complex diagnostic procedures. There seems to be an increase in the incidence of thromboembolic phenomena, probably related to more complex therapeutic procedures and changes in the incidence of diseases since the advent of the antibiotic agents.

This book on venous pressure is intended for beginners in medicine, although it should interest all physicians, especially those entering various cardiovascular fields. The book is not intended to be encyclopedic nor complex. An effort was made to simplify fundamental hemodynamic and cardiovascular principles for the reader. Only fundamental and accepted concepts which are related to venous pressure are presented. The discussion and supporting illustrations are ultimately concerned with venous pressure as related to clinical practice. It is not possible to practice satisfactory cardiology and manage peripheral vascular diseases without a thorough understanding of venous pressure in man in both health and disease. It is hoped that this book provides its readers with such understanding.

I wish to acknowledge the excellent assistance of Miss Ruth Ziifle and Miss Juanita Arbour in my work. The cooperation and assistance of Charles C Thomas, Publisher, in the publication of the monograph is also gratefully acknowledged.

George Burch, M.D.

New Orleans, 1972

CONTENTS

Chapter 1

FUNCTIONAL ANATOMY

Chapter 2

PHYSIOLOGIC CHARACTERISTICS AND HEMODYNAMIC PHENOMENA OF THE CIRCULATION IN VEINS

CHAPTER 3

MEASUREMENT OF VENOUS PRESSURE

CHAPTER 4

NORMAL VALUES OF VENOUS PRESSURE

CHAPTER 5

THE VENOUS PRESSURE IN CERTAIN ABNORMAL CLINICAL STATES

CHAPTER 1

FUNCTIONAL ANATOMY

CERTAIN aspects of the anatomy of veins are of clinical importance for a proper understanding of venous pressure. Some of these aspects have been chosen for illustration with the objective of correlating venous function with venous structure. Many other aspects may suggest themselves to the clinician during the course of observing venous pressure. It will become evident that morphologic development evolves to insure adequate and efficient function.

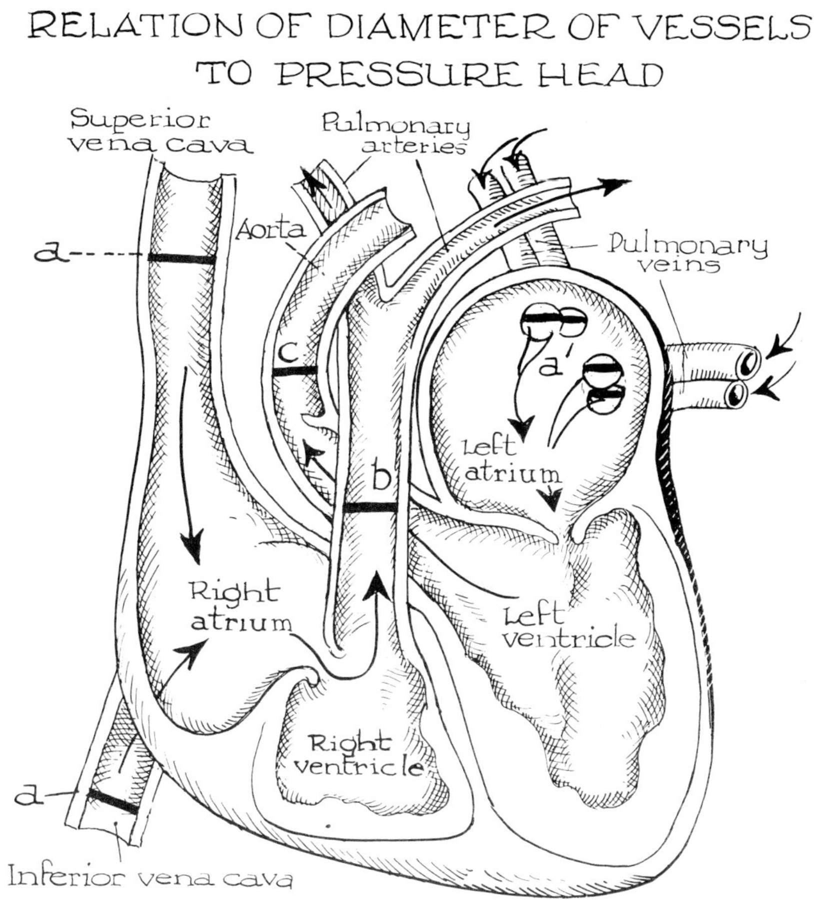

FIG. 1.—Relationship of volume of flow in veins and arteries to their size. The combined diameters or cross-sectional area of the vena cavæ or of the orifices of the pulmonary veins are greater than the diameter of the pulmonary artery or of the aorta. These diameters are indicated by the heavy lines *a*, *a′*, *b*, and *c*.

GENERAL GROSS ANATOMIC FEATURES

Veins are thin-walled vascular tubes which carry blood from the tissues to the heart. Thick muscular walls are not necessary because the pressure within veins is not high. Since the average velocity of flow in veins is less than that in the arteries, since the rate of *volume* flow into the heart is equal to the outflow, and since the arteries and veins tend to parallel each other in length, the veins must have a larger volume and diameter or cross-

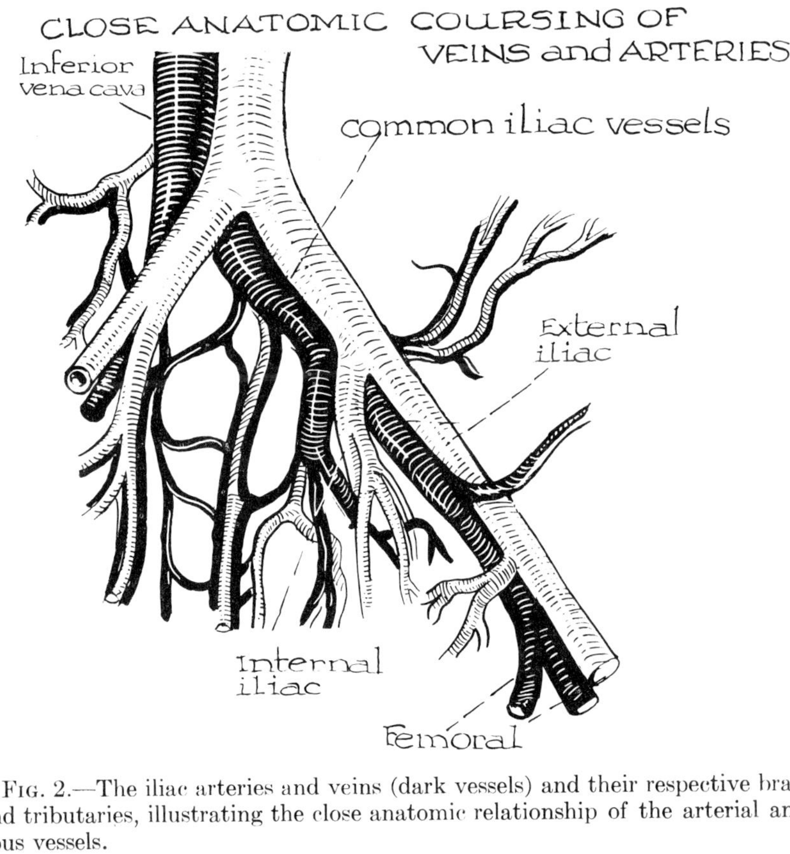

FIG. 2.—The iliac arteries and veins (dark vessels) and their respective branches and tributaries, illustrating the close anatomic relationship of the arterial and venous vessels.

sectional area (Fig. 1). These and other related hemodynamic principles are discussed in greater detail in Chapter 2. The veins, because of their large volume and great extensibility, serve as a reservoir for blood. They tend to course with the arteries, the blood flowing rapidly (linearly) away from the heart in arteries and returning relatively sluggishly (linearly) to it. In general there are two veins to every artery. A typical anatomic relationship of the two groups of vessels is illustrated by Figure 2. Details of nomenclature and description of each vein with its course may be found in textbooks of anatomy and will not be presented here.

The venous system begins at the capillaries and arteriovenous shunts in the tissues. The total cross-sectional area of the veins progressively decreases as the heart is approached and the various tributaries empty into their respective larger collecting veins, the entire venous system, except for the veins of the heart, finally ending in the superior and inferior vena cavae (Fig. 3). Since the volume of blood flowing past any one point of the

VARIATIONS IN VENOUS VOLUME AND CROSS-SECTIONAL AREA

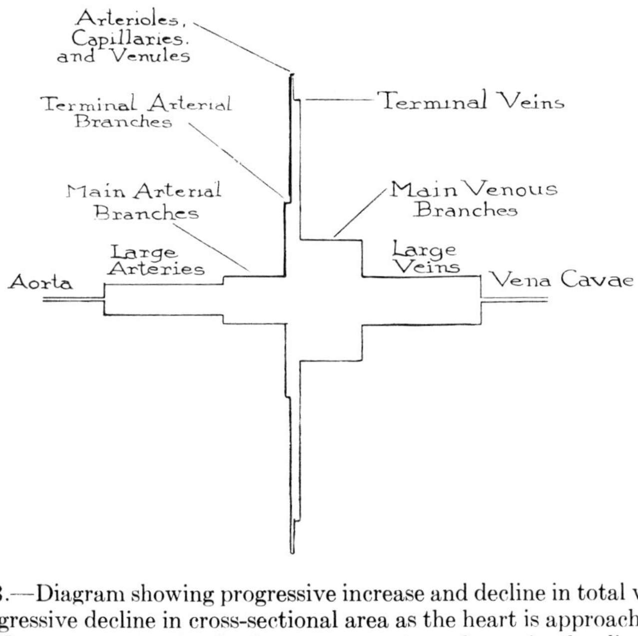

FIG. 3.—Diagram showing progressive increase and decline in total venous volume and progressive decline in cross-sectional area as the heart is approached. Since the volume flow past any point in the venous system shown in the diagram is equal, the linear rate of flow is inversely related to the cross-sectional area at that point. The enclosed area in the diagram is a quantitative index of volume and the transverse diameters of cross-sectional area. Conditions for the arterial side are shown for comparison.

venous system at any one time is essentially the same, with the subject at rest, the linear rate of flow at any one point in the system shown in Figure 3 is inversely related to the cross-sectional area. For example, the linear rate of flow is greater in the vena cavae than in the large veins considered collectively or individually. Therefore, the linear rate of flow in general increases from the periphery to the heart. Since the blood in the veins flows ultimately to the heart and since the blood flows from a point of higher pressure to one of lower pressure, the pressure within the veins must decrease progressively as the heart is approached (Fig. 4 *A*). Furthermore, as the venules and smaller veins empty into larger vessels, the surface area of the veins decreases, so that it is relatively small when the vena cavae are reached (Fig. 4 *B*).

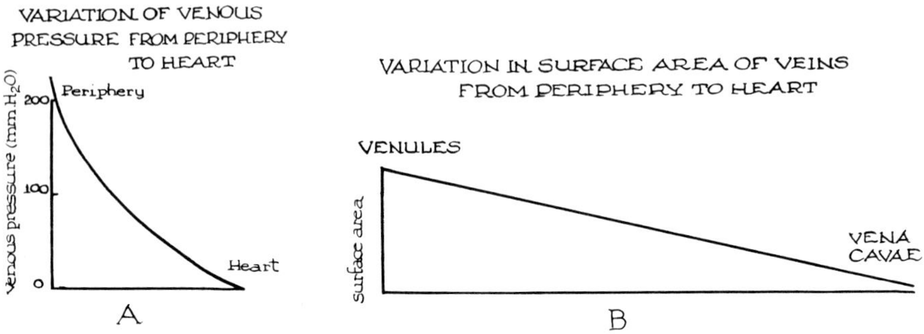

FIG. 4.—*A*, The pressure within and *B*, surface area per unit length of vein decrease as the heart is approached.

The morphologic development of the veins is such as to insure a relatively steady flow of blood to the heart and to maintain a rate of return equal to that required for the cardiac output to supply the tissues with adequate blood to meet the extremes in metabolic demand. This must be done under conditions of wide variations in bodily activity, posture, flexion of parts, intrathoracic pressure, and blood supply to different parts and organs. The anatomic configuration of veins in every detail assists in the performance of these functions, even though considerable variations in structure are necessary from one portion of the body to another. These structural characteristics, which make possible uniform and adequate venous flow, are evident in microscopic and macroscopic details.

MICROSCOPIC ANATOMIC FEATURES

Veins have thinner walls and tend to have larger lumina than arteries (Fig. 5). The relative thinness of the venous wall is attributable to the smaller amount of smooth muscle and collagenous fibers, the veins consisting mainly of connective tissue. For this reason they are flabby or pliable and collapse almost completely when emptied of blood. Like arteries, veins have three main layers (Fig. 6): (1) intima, (2) media, and (3) adventitia. The structure of the layers of a medium-sized vein is essentially as follows:

1) The **intima** is composed of thin or flat cells which are short and polygonal in shape. Their longitudinal axis is perpendicular to the predominant direction of the longitudinal axis of the smooth muscle in the wall of the vein. These cells are said to have phagocytic ability. The endothelium provides a smooth lining which reduces friction to flowing blood and is also "wetted" by the blood; it has certain functions concerned with preventing intravenous clotting. The endothelium is "folded" at selected points to form valves, which are discussed in greater detail later.

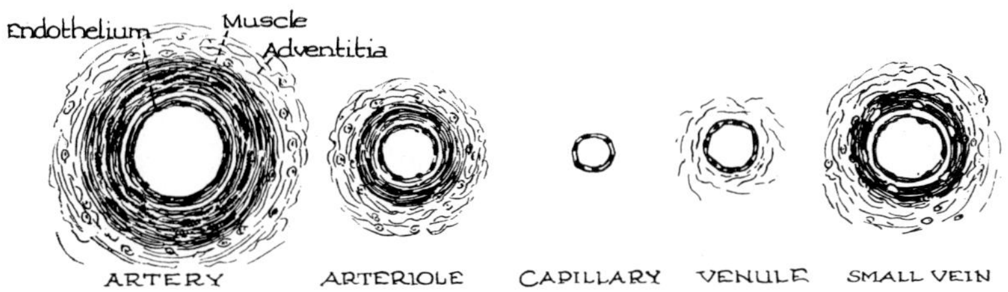

Fig. 5.—Microscopic appearance of a small artery, arteriole, capillary, venule and small vein.

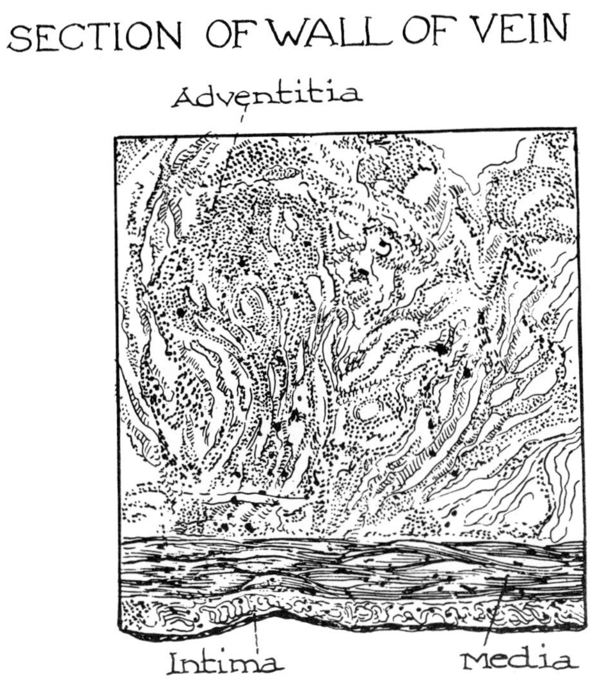

Fig. 6.—Microscopic appearance of a transverse section through the wall of a large vein.

The subendothelial layer (Fig. 6), which consists of delicate elastic and collagenous fibers, is more highly developed in the larger veins and is absent in the extremely small ones. These fibers course spirally and longitudinally and vary in amount in different veins.

2) The **media** of veins is much thinner in comparison to that of arterioles of equal luminal size. It consists of elastic and collagenous fibers which are intermingled with circular smooth muscle. In the larger veins the muscle tends to be gathered in bundles with the intervening elastic and collagenous connective tissue. The media is thicker in the vessels of the lower extremities and almost absent in those of the head and neck. In certain sharply localized areas, the muscle thickens to form functioning sphincters.

3) The **adventitia** is highly developed and constitutes the greater portion of the venous wall. It consists of an abundance of elastic and collagenous fibers of connective tissue and muscular bundles which course longitudinally. Like the others, this largest layer varies in degree of development, being highly developed in the inferior vena cava and other veins of the abdomen, such as the portal vein, and almost lacking in the thoracic veins, such as the superior vena cava, azygos and innominate.

SPECIAL FUNCTIONAL ANATOMIC CHARACTERISTICS

Although veins consist of three layers, variations in histologic characteristics are considerable and the layers are not sharply demarcated, one blending into another. Veins that support relatively high pressure, such as those of the lower extremities, have thicker walls with more collagenous tissue and smooth muscle. In general, walls of veins of equal luminal size are of essentially the same thickness in the same organs. Even though the pressure within the veins decreases from the periphery to the heart, the diameter of the individual vessels increases. The force against the wall is

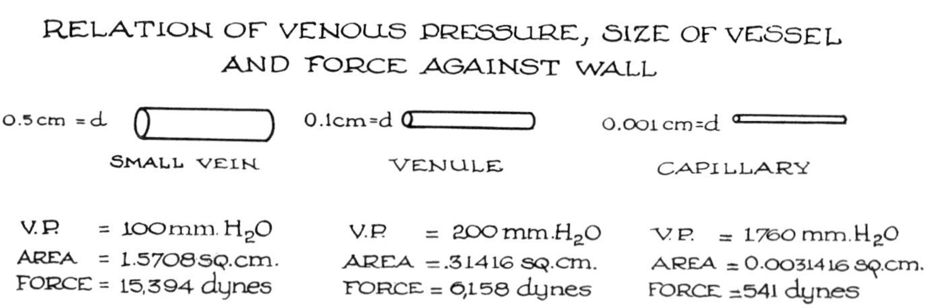

FIG. 7.—Force on the wall of the more peripheral veins is less than that on the more central ones because of the smaller surface area per unit of length of vein. The variables are indicated in the illustration.

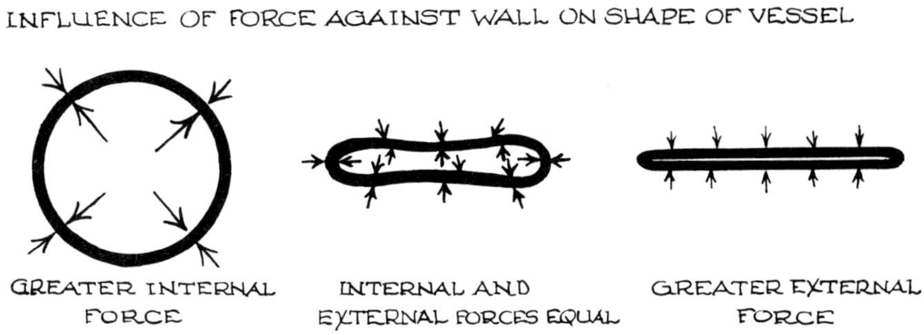

FIG. 8.—Influence of internal and external forces on shape and form of veins.

proportional to the surface area. Although the pressure is greater in the more peripheral veins, the force supported by a unit length of vein is less than that on the more central ones (Fig. 7), and therefore the walls of the more peripheral veins would be expected to be thinner (Fig. 5). The force on a unit length of vein increases in amount from the periphery to the heart even though the pressure decreases, because the surface area upon which the pressure acts increases as the diameter of the vein increases (Fig. 7).

Because veins are flabby and pliable, they collapse readily when emptied of blood, indicating that their state of distention in the body is dependent upon the difference in internal and external forces acting upon them (Fig. 8). Arterial configuration is less influenced by external forces encountered in the body. Organic structure, traction by organs such as the lungs, pressure within the tissues and many other factors influencing extravenous

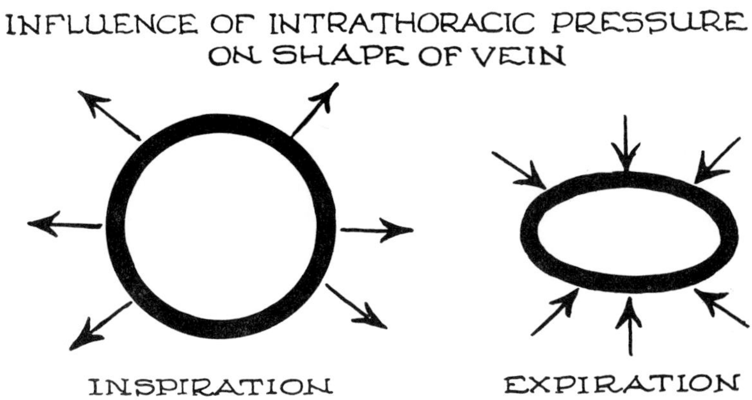

FIG. 9.—Influence of negative and relatively low positive thoracic pressure upon the patency and shape of intrathoracic veins.

pressure affect the size and form of the venous lumina. The negative pressure during inspiration and slightly positive pressure during expiration vary the external forces on the veins in the thorax from moment to moment and, therefore, the net force acting upon the walls of the veins from within. The net influence of the relatively low intrathoracic pressure acting externally is to maintain patency of the thoracic veins (Fig. 9). On the other hand, the relatively high positive intra-abdominal pressure tends to exert an external force upon the intra-abdominal veins which tends to collapse them. This force is overcome in part by fairly thick layers of longitudinal elastic and muscular fibers found in the walls of the large intra-abdominal veins, such as the inferior vena cava, which assist the internal venous pressure in maintaining patency of the vessel (Fig. 10). In addition, the longi-

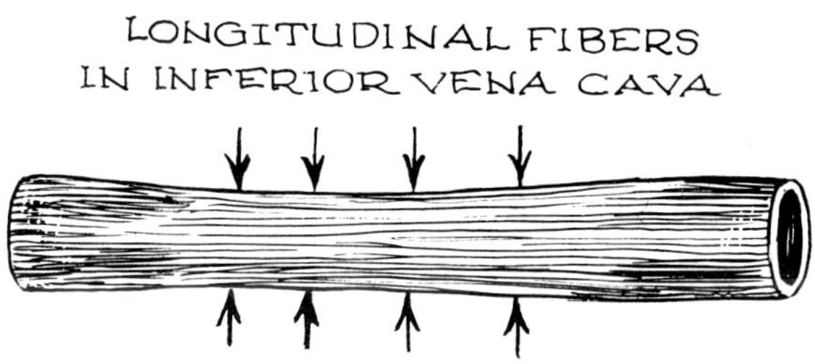

FIG. 10.—The longitudinal elastic and muscular fibers tend to keep the inferior vena cavæ open in spite of the positive intra-abdominal pressure.

tudinal fibers allow the inferior vena cava to shorten and lengthen as the diaphragm moves cephalad and caudad during expiration and inspiration.

The *collagenous fibers,* which are loose and wavy, form a *spiral network* in the walls of the veins. These characteristics permit the veins to dilate readily, so that a relatively large volume of blood may be accommodated with only a slight rise in venous pressure. *Circular fibers* are found in greater number in vessels with high venous pressure.

Smooth muscle is highly developed in veins with high pressure and in areas where sphincteric function is necessary. The veins of the pregnant uterus and adrenal glands are rich in smooth muscle, whereas others, like the retinal veins, veins of the dura and pia mater, sinuses of erectile tissue, veins of the nail bed, and "giant capillaries" of the skin, are devoid of muscle.

SUPPLY OF NERVES TO THE VEINS

The veins, like the arteries, are supplied by the sympathetic nervous system. Afferent medullated nerves reach the veins from essentially the same centers as those which supply the arterial side of the circulation, but the former has not received the attention of the arterial system. Neural fibers envelop adventitial cells and muscles of the media (Fig. 11). Each muscular cell appears to be innervated separately. The veins contain receptor end-organs which include arborization and Pacinian corpuscles. In general, the veins respond to the same type of stimuli, mediated through

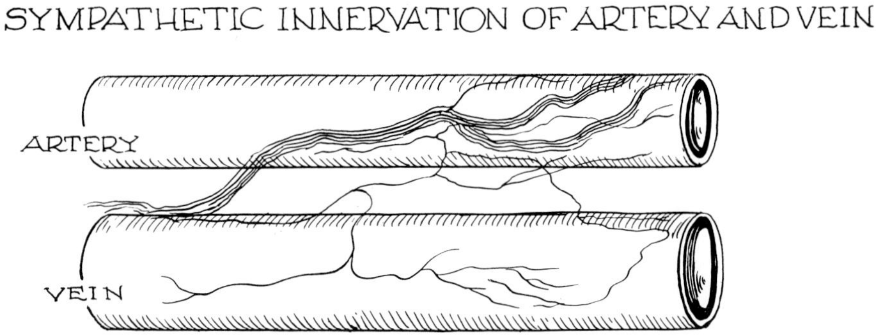

FIG. 11.—Diagram of sympathetic innervation of a vein.

the sympathetic nervous system, as do the arteries and arterioles. Since the same principles of innervation and function of the autonomic system can be applied to veins as to arteries and since those of the latter are so well known, such details will not be included in these discussions except under special circumstances.

The importance of the smooth muscles and nerves in the wall of the veins becomes evident when it is remembered that the venous system is a large dynamic reservoir or pool in which blood can be placed into more active or less active circulation to meet emergencies associated with sudden variations in blood volume or volume of the vascular bed. When the veins contract, thereby momentarily accelerating the rate of return of blood to the heart and also causing a shift of venous blood to the large vessels near the heart initiating the Bainbridge reflex, cardiac output increases. The nervous system permits coordination of the entire venous system. Shortly following sympathectomy venous tone is regained, and the smooth muscle of the veins comes under the control of local stimuli and circulating chemical factors.

THE VASA VASORUM

The veins are richly supplied with vasa vasorum (Fig. 12), to a greater extent than are the arteries. Even those 1 mm. in diameter receive a blood supply within their walls. There is no evidence that vasa vasorum connect with the lumen of the veins, although they penetrate to the subintimal layers. The media is richly supplied. There is a well developed anastamosis of the vasa vasorum within the walls of the veins. Although nourishment for the veins is derived from these vessels, nutrient materials diffuse directly through the endothelial lining of the veins, which is, of course, the important source of foodstuffs in the smallest veins deprived of vasa vasorum.

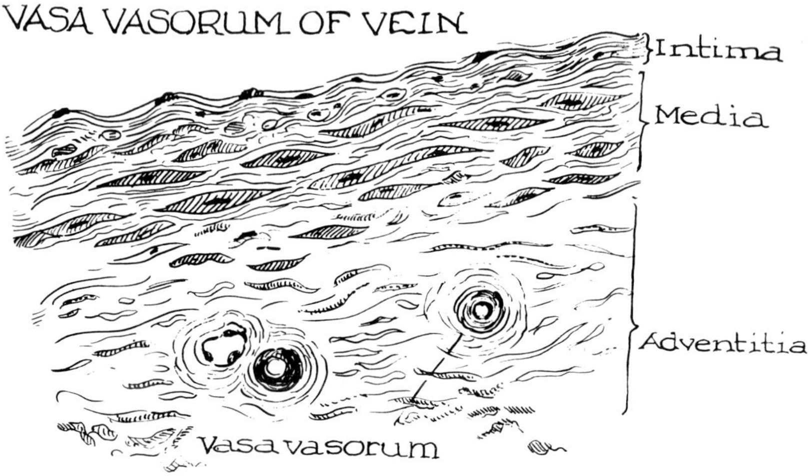

FIG. 12.—Vasa vasorum within a segment of the wall of a vein.

VALVES OF VEINS

The physiologic importance of valves in veins is well known to all clinicians. They develop early in fetal life in relatively large numbers, many never reaching complete development, and recede as the fetus grows. After birth the number of valves decreases with age. The number in the upper portions of the body is much greater during fetal life than at the time of birth. The significance of the changes with growth and the function of valves *in utero* are unknown.

Venous valves represent reflection of the intima of veins (Fig. 13). The valves are composed of leaflets, varying in number from one to three, and rarely four. They are called, accordingly, unicuspid, bicuspid, and tricuspid (Fig. 15). Veins of narrow caliber usually have unicuspid valves, whereas large veins have bicuspid or, less frequently, tricuspid valves.

The valvular leaflets form *semilunar cusps*. Bulging and thinning of the wall of the veins proximal to the valves form sinuses which are opposite the valvular cusps (Fig. 14). The sinuses and valvular cusps are directed

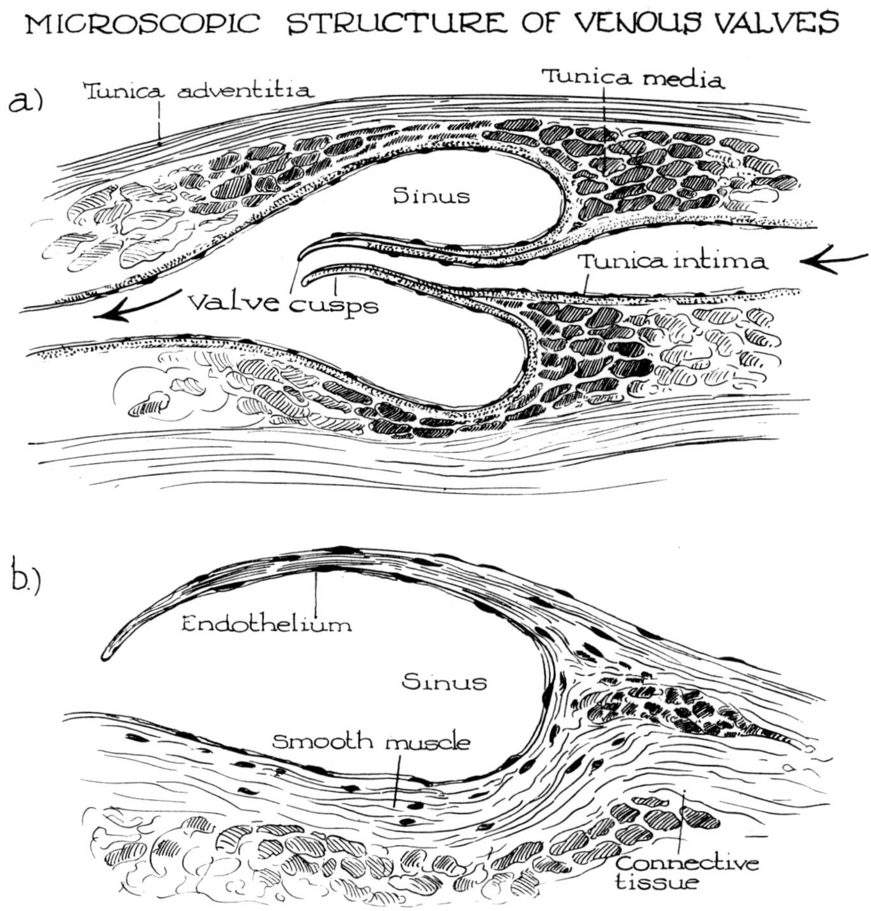

FIG. 13.—Longitudinal microscopic section through a vein and valve.

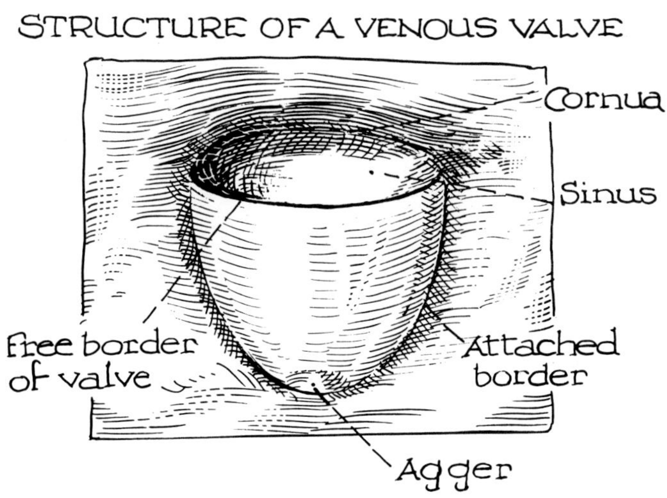

FIG. 14.—A segment of vein opened to show the structure of an intact venous valve.

toward the heart or in the direction of blood flow in the vein except in some of the veins of the head (page 25). Structural details of a venous valve are shown in Figure 14.

Microscopic Characteristics.—The *valve* is a thin pliable leaflet composed of a reflection of the endothelium of the vein. The endothelial cells on the surface of the valve facing the lumen of the vein course longitudinally or parallel with the longitudinal axis of the vein; the longitudinal axis of the

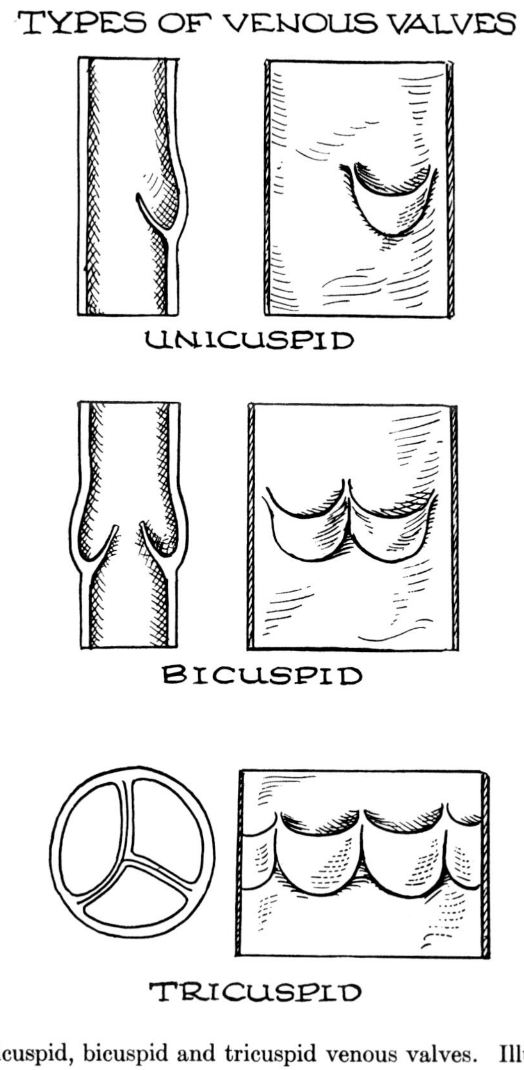

FIG. 15.—Unicuspid, bicuspid and tricuspid venous valves. Illustrations on the left are cross sections through the valves; those on the right show the internal surface of the vein.

endothelial cells covering the surface of valve facing the sinuses course transversely. There is a thin, loose network of elastic fibers within the leaflet between the two endothelial surfaces. In the immediate region of the valve at its base and at the sinus where the wall of the vein is thin.

Distribution of Venous Valves in the Adult.—There are no valves in the venous sinuses of the head and neck, including the tributaries of the ophthalmic, meningeal, and cerebral veins. The emissary veins joining the superior sagittal sinus, the veins of the diploe and of the scalp possess *valves directed peripherally*. Thus, the relative direction and local morphologic characteristics tend to vary according to their position with respect to the heart.

The tributaries of the internal jugular, facial, lingual, superior thyroid, and temporal veins possess valves at their orifices. At the lower end of the *jugular bulb* there is usually a unicuspid, bicuspid or tricuspid valve. A unicuspid or bicuspid valve usually occurs at the entrance of the deep *cervical vein* into the vertebral vein. The *anterior jugular vein* has no valves, whereas the *external jugular* usually has an incompetent one near its junction with the subclavian and one just about 2.5 to 5 cm. above the clavicle. There are many valves in the veins of the upper limbs, especially in the deep veins. Although the *innominate vein* has no valves, the orifices of its tributaries are guarded by them. The *subclavian vein* has at least one valve located just before its junction with the *external jugular vein*. The *internal mammary veins* and their tributaries possess valves, but the *azygos* and *hemiazygos* have only incompetent ones. At the orifices of the *intercostal veins* they also occur, but there are none in the venous plexuses of the vertebral column and spinal cord, except at the exits of the main channels.

There are no valves in the veins of the *thoracic viscera*, but they may occur at the termination of the *cardiac veins*. The *great cardiac vein* is guarded at its mouth by the bicuspid valvula Vieussenii, which is present in young persons and is retained in a less prominent state in about 80 per cent of adults. With growth many of the valves in coronary veins are lost.

The entrance of the *hepatic* vein into the inferior vena cava is guarded not by the usual type of venous valve but rather by a sickle-shaped fold and "sluice" valve, which appears to vary considerably in development with individuals. The veins of the *abdominal viscera* have valves, but those of the *renal veins* are rudimentary. Though the *common iliac* and *hypogastric veins* rarely possess valves, their tributaries do. About 35 per cent of the *external iliac veins* possess valves, most of which are not fully developed. The veins of the *lower extremities* are well supplied with them, and these are almost without exception bicuspid.

"**Venous Pumps**".—There are no valves in the veins within the muscles but they do exist immediately at the point where the veins exit from the muscles and enter the larger collecting veins. In such a specific location these valves make "venous pumps" possible (Fig. 16). The first part of Figure 16 shows a relaxed muscle. When the muscle relaxes, the venous pressure in the veins located within the muscle declines and the valve (*a*) just external to the muscle closes, preventing the intramuscular veins from refilling from the large collecting veins external to the muscle. Instead, the veins within the muscle refill from the arterial system supplying the muscle. Valve (*b*) in the extramuscular collecting vein and located distal to the entrance of

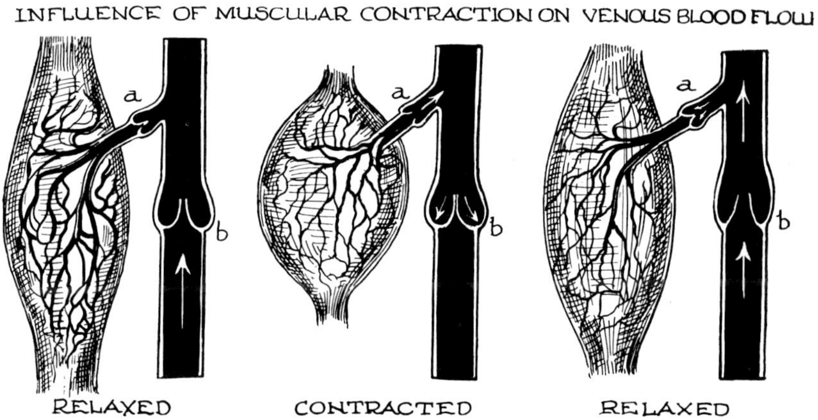

FIG. 16.—Diagram showing the function of a valve at exit of a vein from a muscle. Consult the text for details.

the vein from the muscle is closed if the pressure proximal to it is higher than that distally. It is open, however, when the pressure distally is higher. The second part of Figure 16 shows a contracted muscle. Valve (*a*) opens as the intramuscular tissue pressure squeezes upon the walls of the intramuscular veins to raise the venous pressure within them to a level which is higher than that in the extramuscular collecting vein. Blood is, therefore, forced out through valve (*a*) into the collecting veins and toward the heart. Valve (*b*) is closed if the pressure proximal to it is elevated to a level above that in the venous segment distal to this valve. This is likely to happen with sudden and strong contractions of the muscle. As blood flows toward the heart, the pressure proximal to valve (*b*) declines, the pressure distal to it again becomes higher, and valve (*b*) reopens, so that blood flows toward the heart from peripheral tissues (last part of Fig. 16).

It does not require a great deal of imagination to visualize the mechanism and movement of these important, rapidly and passively functioning venous valves. Their location and function among the muscles of the body insure unidirectional flow of blood toward the heart and make possible the venous pumps.

Special Types of Venous Valves.—(*1*) The *"sluice valve"* at the point of entrance of the hepatic vein into the inferior vena cava is aided by a semilunar fold of endothelium (Fig. 17), which prevents regurgitation of

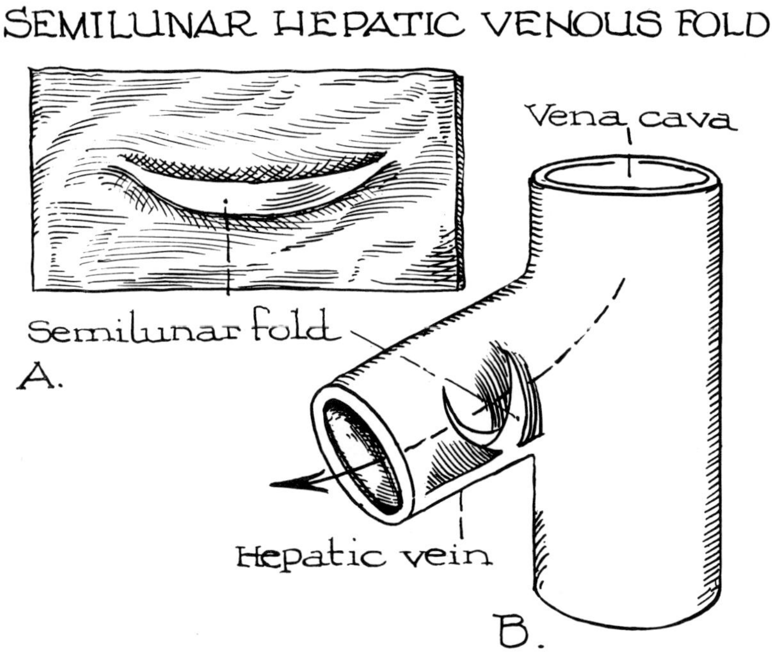

FIG. 17.—A segment of hepatic vein opened *A*, to show the intact semilunar fold guarding the entrance of the hepatic vein into the inferior vena cava. *B* is a three dimensional diagram showing the sickle-shaped or semilunar fold.

blood from the inferior vena cava into the liver, as might occur during coughing, speaking, defecation, or any other action accompanied by sudden increase in pressure within the vena cava. The sluice valve at the entrance of the hepatic vein into the inferior vena cava is activated by a relatively thick mass of longitudinal smooth muscular fibers in the wall of the inferior vena cava which loop around the inferior aspect of the hepatic vein as it penetrates the wall of the inferior vena cava (Fig. 18). When these muscular fibers contract, the inferior semicircular portion of the orifice and semilunar fold of the hepatic vein are elevated, thus narrowing the portal of entrance of the hepatic vein into the inferior vena cava (Fig. 18). When these muscular fibers relax, the elastic fibers of connective tissue within the wall of the vein pull the inferior portion of the hepatic vein at its orifice caudad, enlarging the orifice and reducing resistance to the flow of blood into the inferior vena cava (Fig. 18). The semilunar fold aids in the function of the sluice valve. These structures are highly developed in some animals but poorly developed in man. The anatomic and physiologic circumstances in man have been little studied.

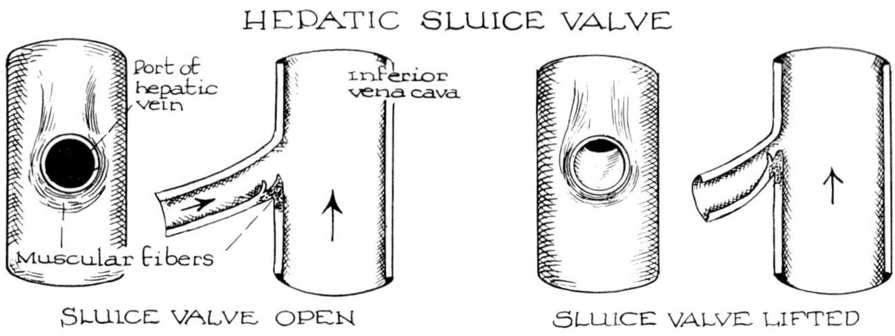

FIG. 18.—Action of the sluice valve at the entrance of the inferior vena cava. Consult text for details of action.

2) *Flutter valves* exist proximal to the point of entrance of some veins into a large collecting vein (Fig. 19). Their function is simple and, of course, is passive. This type of valve is highly developed in the horse.

3) *Sphincters* sometimes develop to aid in the control of the direction of flow of venous blood; these consist of a local increase in the amount of circular smooth muscle at the entrance of a tributary into a collecting vein. Such a sphincter is seen at the orifice of the renal vein (Fig. 20). A special type of sphincteric action occurs at the entrance of the superior and inferior vena cavae into the right atrium. It is produced by a reflection of the right atrial cardiac muscle onto the vena cavae for a short distance (Fig. 21). When atrial contraction occurs, this general area contracts first, narrowing the portal of the vena cavae and limiting the amount of blood which can regurgitate from the right atrium into the vena cavae. A flow into the right ventricle, or unidirectional flow, is therefore insured. These venous sphincters are highly developed in lower animals and are more highly developed in the human fetus than in the adult, since they decrease in number and atrophy to some extent with growth and aging.

Antigravitational Function of Venous Valves.—The valves in veins have an antigravitational function, which is manifested best in the lower extremities, where the column of blood in a standing man is long and where, therefore, the pressure is great. When a person suddenly stands, a large pressure or force of the long column of blood is thrown at once upon the

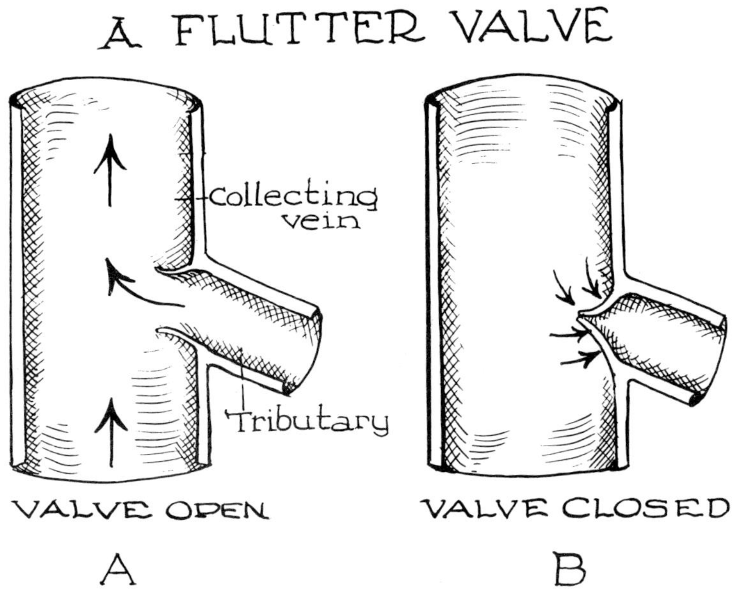

FIG. 19.—A "flutter valve" at entrance of a tributary into a collecting vein. *A* shows valve partially open, since pressure in the tributary is slightly greater than in the collecting vein. *B* show the valve closed, as pressure is now higher in the collecting vein.

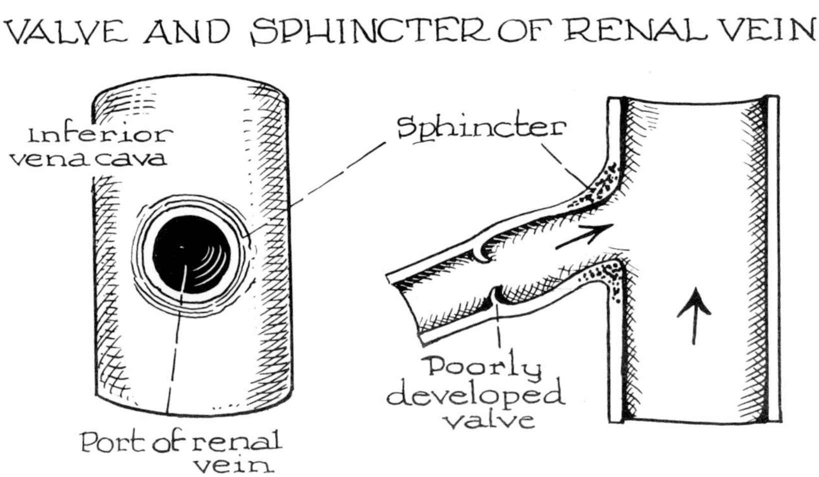

FIG. 20.—Sphincter of smooth muscle at port of renal vein.

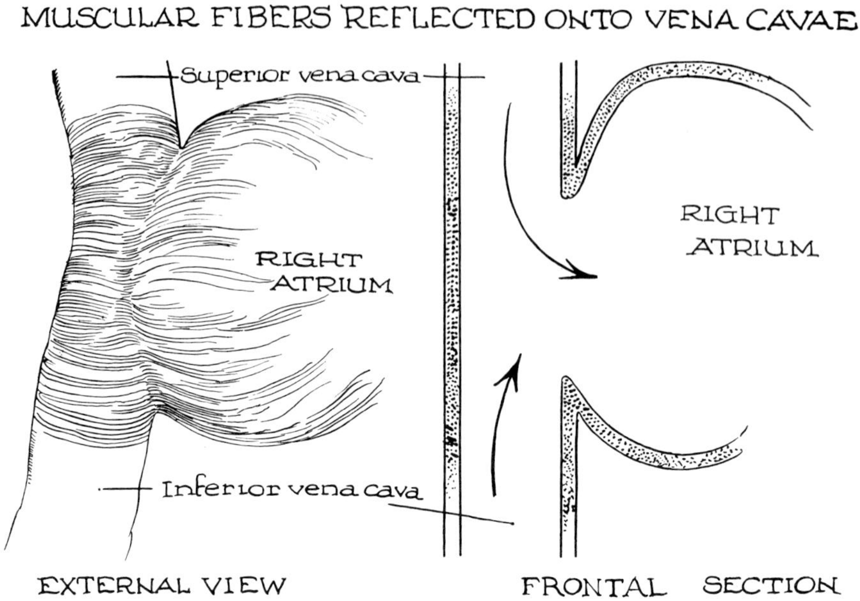

FIG. 21.—Sphincter of reflected cardiac muscle around the vena cavæ near the entrance of the superior and inferior vena cavæ into the right atrium.

veins of the legs. Because of the large number of valves in the veins of these limbs, this column is immediately broken into small segments as the person stands, and the degree of force suddenly thrust upon any segment of vein is consequently reduced (Fig. 22).

Figure 22 illustrates diagrammatically the action of venous valves in overcoming the effects of gravity. With the vein horizontal (Fig. 22 *A*), as in a lower extremital vein of a man resting supine, gravity has practically no effect on intravenous pressure. If he were suddenly to stand erect and if there were no valves in the veins, the force or weight of the entire column of blood would fall upon the wall of the vein and would increase progressively as the distal end was approached (Fig. 22 *B*). However, since the valves break the column into small segments when the subject stands, each segment would sustain a relatively small amount of pressure (Fig. 22 *C*). Should the man remain erect, blood would be continually delivered by the arteries to the limbs distal to the valves. This blood would gradually accumulate and its pressure would rise progressively until the pressure distal to each valve became greater than that proximal to the valve. When this happens, the valves would open and the circulation would be re-established with the full pressure or force of the column of blood being lodged against the wall of the vein (Fig. 22 *D*).

The antigravitational role of valves protects such organs as the liver, kidneys, and gastrointestinal tract, in addition to tissues of the limbs. The function of these anatomic structures prevents sudden hemodynamic disturbances with sudden changes in posture.

Extent of Opening of Venous Valves.—The extent to which the valves are opened is determined by the rate of flow of blood through them. With rapid flow the valves tend to open wider, whereas at extremely slow rates they are only slightly patent. As the blood flows around the edges of the

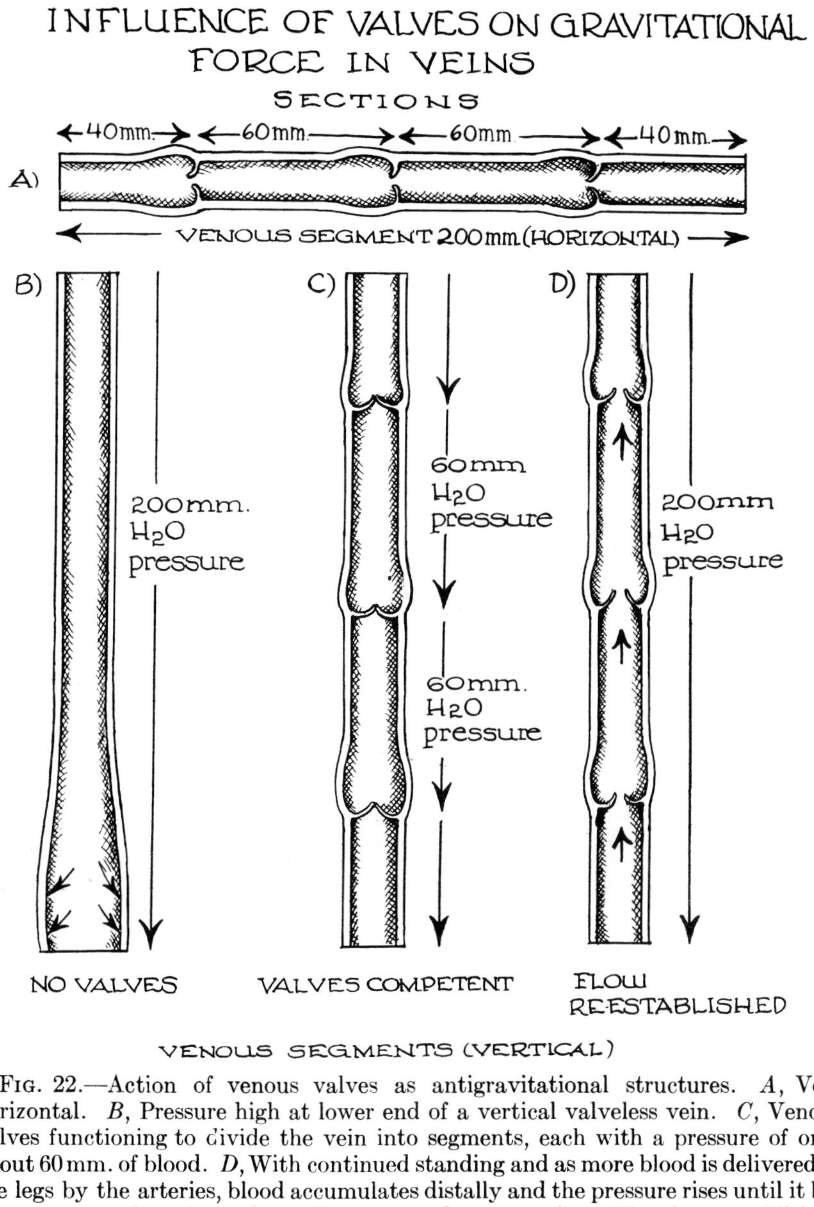

FIG. 22.—Action of venous valves as antigravitational structures. *A*, Vein horizontal. *B*, Pressure high at lower end of a vertical valveless vein. *C*, Venous valves functioning to divide the vein into segments, each with a pressure of only about 60 mm. of blood. *D*, With continued standing and as more blood is delivered to the legs by the arteries, blood accumulates distally and the pressure rises until it becomes greater than the hydrostatic pressure due to gravity. Flow is re-established.

valves, eddy currents are formed, which tend to keep them projected into the lumen of the vein. These partially closed valves are readily shut—almost immediately—when the direction of flow of blood begins to reverse (Fig. 23).

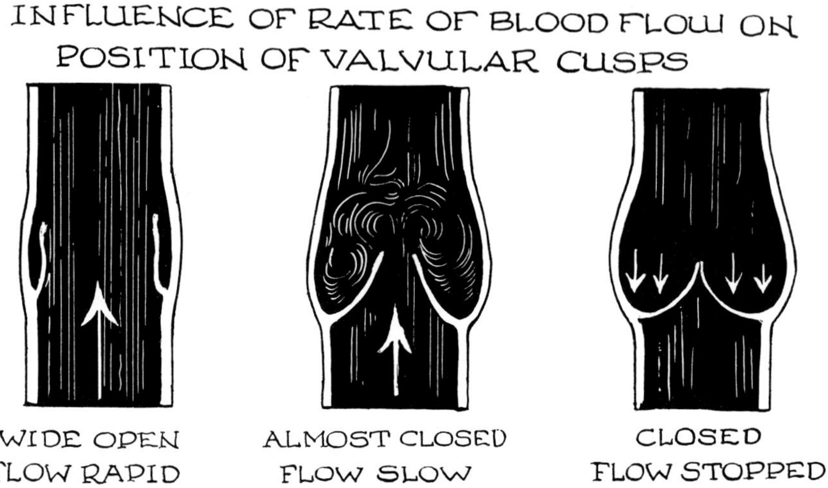

FIG. 23.—Venous valve opened relatively wide during rapid flow, partially opened and held ajar by eddy currents and the flowing blood during slow flow, and closed when the direction of flow tends to be reversed.

In most instances, small tributaries which empty into large collecting veins are guarded by valves near the point of communication (Fig. 24). This permits considerable variation in pressure within the large vein without regurgitation of blood into the tributary.

The function of venous valves is influenced by local venous tone. When the tone is reduced or when there is local venous dilatation, the consequent

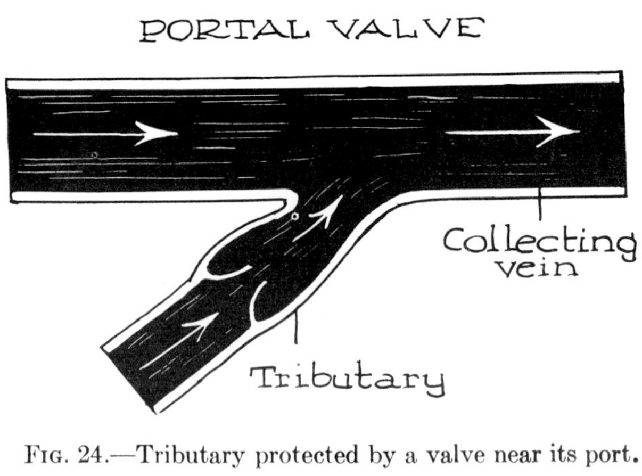

FIG. 24.—Tributary protected by a valve near its port.

increase in diameter of the vein makes it impossible for the valves to bridge the lumen completely, so that valvular incompetency ensues (Fig. 25). With increase in tone, the veins narrow and valvular competency is re-established (Fig. 25). Venous dilatation and valvular incompetency may occur in an extremely warm environment; in a cool environment venous tone is increased, the lumen narrows, and the valves are competent.

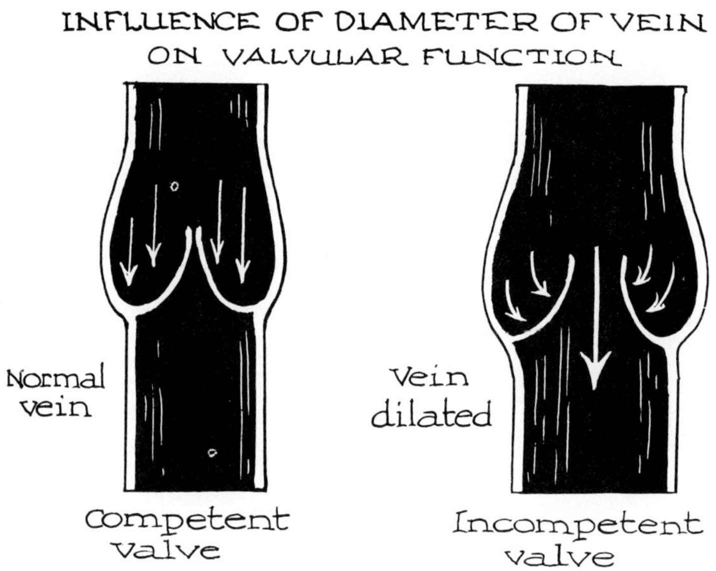

FIG. 25.—Influence of diameter of the vein on the function of venous valves.

SPECIFIC VEINS

Veins of the Arms and Neck.—The walls of the veins of the *upper extremities* are not as thick as those of the lower extremities because, as a result of gravity, they are not normally subjected to as high venous pressure as those of the legs. The *jugular* and other *veins of the neck* also have thin walls, since the pressure within them is low. The larger veins of the upper portions of the body contain the layers and general characteristics previously described for veins in general.

Near the entrance of the *superior vena cava* into the right atrium there is a thin layer of cardiac muscle (Fig. 21). Relatively thick layers of circular and longitudinal smooth muscle replace the cardiac muscle a few millimeters from the right atrium.

The *pulmonary veins* in the extrapulmonary portions of the thorax contain a thick layer of smooth muscle, whereas those in the intrapulmonary

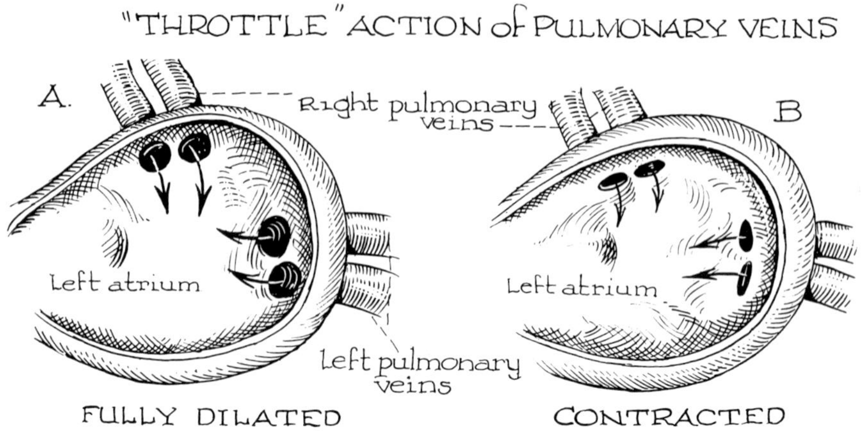

Fig. 26.—"Throttle" action of the pulmonary veins in the control of blood flow to the left atrium. *A*, Pulmonary veins dilated to increase the rate of return of blood. *B*, Pulmonary veins contracted to decrease venous return.

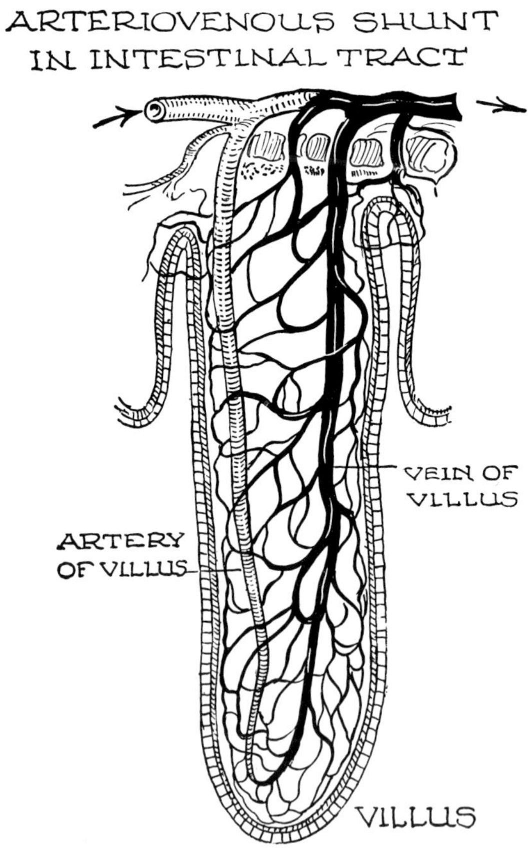

Fig. 27.—Arteriovenous shunting provided by an extremely vascular villus of the jejunum.

portions have less muscle. Striated muscle has been described in the extrapulmonary portions, the quantity being greater in adults than in children. Elastic fibers are numerous. The muscular fibers of the large veins only are supplied with afferent and efferent neural fibers.

The pulmonary veins, and to a lesser extent the hepatic veins, have a "throttle" function or may be considered as "throttle veins" (Fig. 26). A thick layer of smooth muscle accumulates to form sphincters in the region of the orifices of the four pulmonary veins. These sphincters can contract or dilate in order to increase or decrease the rate of flow of blood to the left side of the heart (Fig. 26). The extent to which these are developed in man is unknown but they may be important clinically.

Portal Vein.—The numerous small vessels of the submucosal layer of the intestinal tract, especially of the villi, act as arteriovenous shunts. There are also direct arteriovenous shunts which make it possible for blood of the mesenteric arterial system to be shunted directly into the portal venous system (Fig. 27). By means of these direct shunts arterial blood is delivered straight into the portal venous system without first entering the villi. Such direct connections, as well as the many indirect ones, permit transmission of pressure from the heart and arterial system into the portal venous system. This *vis a tergo* is of considerable importance in maintaining the portal venous pressure and portal circulation through the liver.

DISTENSIBILITY OF VEINS

As stated previously, the veins may become *distended* by relatively small elevations in venous pressure, due to the loose connective tissue of the venous wall and the thinness of the wall. However, if the pressure in a venous segment is progressively increased until the limits of distensibility are reached, the fibers will be stretched, and the configuration of the molecular complexes forming the connective tissue fibers will be altered. If stretching is not prolonged or if it is not excessive, release of pressure will result in prompt return of the venous wall and luminal size to the previous resting configuration (Fig. 28). However, if the pressure in the vein is increased greatly, the wall will become overstretched and the structural configurations will be distorted to such an extent that the venous wall will remain distorted for a long time after venous pressure has returned to normal (Fig. 28).

Strength of Veins.—Veins are not easily ruptured by venous pressure. The iliac vein of man, like his carotid artery, can withstand a pressure of 7 to 8 atmospheres. The inferior vena cava and femoral vein have been found to be strongest at the age of thirty years.

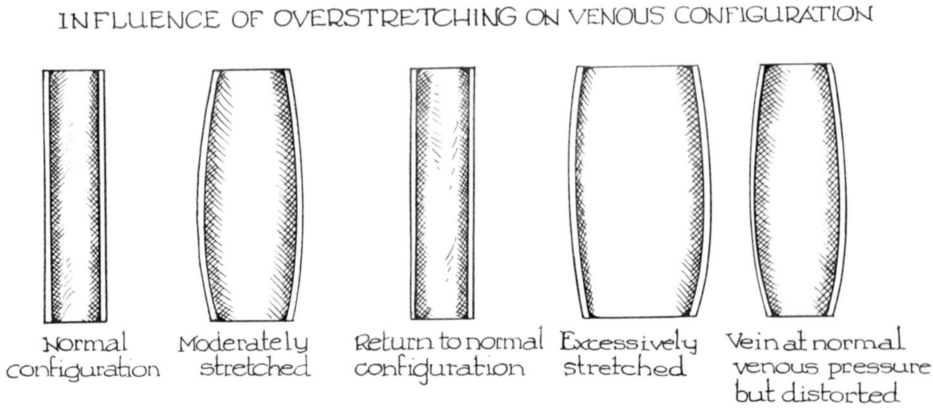

FIG. 28.—Influence of distending and stretching a vein by moderate and great increases in intravenous pressure.

Rigidity of Venous Wall.—As the venous pressure increases, the characteristics of the veins change from those of freely distensible tubes to those of more rigid nondistensible ones (Fig. 29). The stretched wall is relatively firm and turgid, whereas that of the nondistended vein is pliable and flabby. By the standards of the hydraulic engineer, even the wall of distended veins would not approach the rigidity of the wall of iron pipes. The relative pliability of the venous wall is, of course, important in hemodynamics and is partially responsible for differences between the problems in the physics of blood vessels and in those of hydraulic engineering.

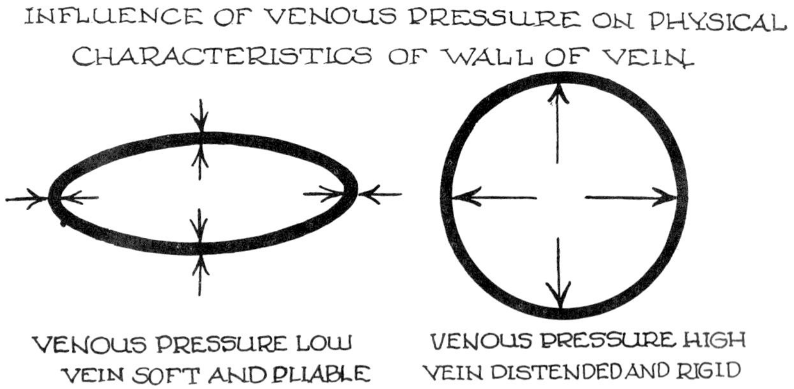

FIG. 29.—At low venous pressure, the venous wall is soft, pliable and flabby; at high venous pressure, the venous wall is firm, rigid and stretched.

CHAPTER 2

PHYSIOLOGIC CHARACTERISTICS AND HEMODYNAMIC PHENOMENA OF THE CIRCULATION IN VEINS

BEFORE a discussion of general physiologic phenomena is undertaken and their clinical applications are approached, it is advisable to consider the hemodynamic principles peculiar to the venous system. It is well to note that although millimeters of water and blood are frequently used interchangeably throughout the text for simplicity, differences due to specific gravity must be considered.

POISEUILLE'S LAW

Nonturbulent flow of fluid through small tubes, such as veins, follows Poiseuille's law (Fig. 30), expressed by the equation

$$Q = \frac{\pi p r^4 t}{8 l \eta}, \qquad (1)$$

where Q is volume of fluid flowing through a tube in time t,
p is the fall in pressure in the direction of flow over the length l,
r is the radius of the tube,
l is the length of the tube, and
η is the coefficient of viscosity.

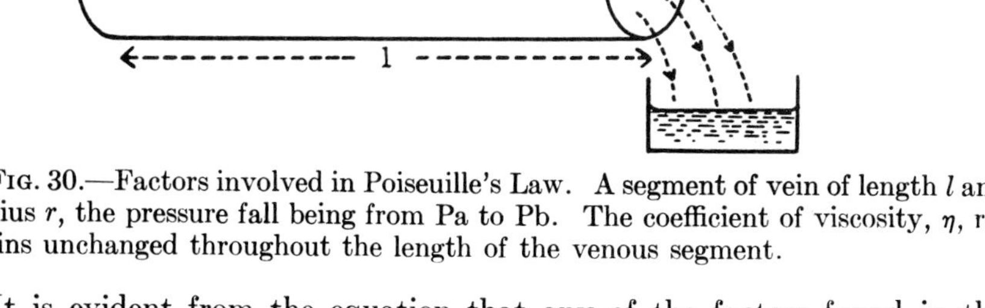

FIG. 30.—Factors involved in Poiseuille's Law. A segment of vein of length *l* and radius *r*, the pressure fall being from Pa to Pb. The coefficient of viscosity, η, remains unchanged throughout the length of the venous segment.

It is evident from the equation that any of the factors found in the numerator of the fraction is directly related to blood flow and any factor in the denominator is inversely related to flow. For example, if a factor in the numerator increases in value, the rate of blood flow increases, whereas an increase in any factor in the denominator is associated with a decrease in blood flow. Because of their importance each factor is discussed in greater detail later.

Before a discussion of the factors concerned with blood flow, as defined by Poiseuille's equation, is undertaken, it is important to note that the equation may be expressed in several ways so as to indicate the manner in which any factor is altered in magnitude by a variation of the other functions. Because these discussions are concerned primarily with venous pressure, it is interesting to write the equation so that pressure, p, is the dependent variable, *i. e.*,

$$p = \frac{8l\eta Q}{\pi r^4 t}. \qquad (2)$$

From inspection of the various independent functions it is easy to note quickly which are directly or inversely related to pressure head. For example, an increase in length of the tube, viscosity of the blood or rate of blood flow would be associated with an increase in pressure head if all other factors remain constant. On the other hand an increase in diameter of the vessel or in time would be associated with a decrease in pressure head if all other factors remain constant. The interrelationship of these factors should become clear with the discussion of the variables immediately following.

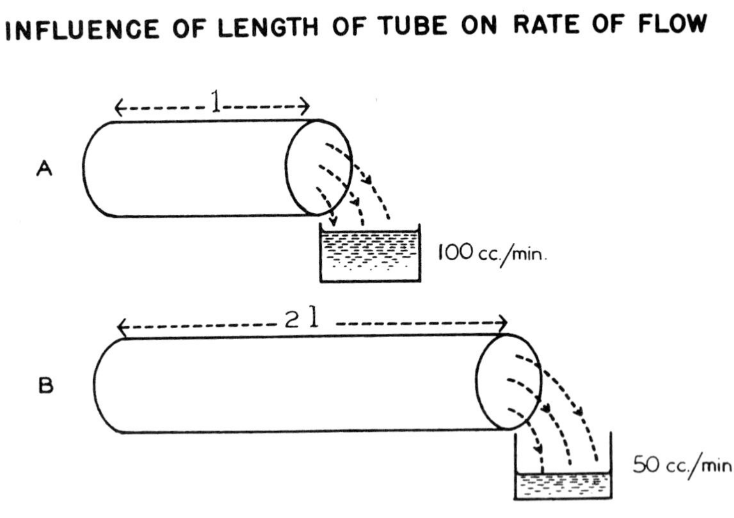

FIG. 31.—If all factors remain unchanged, quantity of blood flowing through a vein of length l, *A*, per unit of time is twice as large as that flowing through a similar vein twice as long, *B*.

Influence of Length of Vein on Rate of Volume Flow.—According to Poiseuille's law, the longer the vein, l, the smaller the quantity of blood that will flow through the vein in a unit of time, everything else being constant. This is evident, since l is a factor in the denominator of the fraction in equation (1). If the length is doubled, the quantity of fluid that will flow through the vein per unit of time will be reduced by one-half (Fig. 31). Therefore, the longer a vein, the more difficult it is for blood to flow through it. This impairment of flow is due to frictional resistance to flow.

Diameter of Vein.—Poiseuille's law indicates that the larger the diameter of the lumen of a vein, the larger is the rate of flow of blood through the vessel; specifically, the volume of blood that flows through a vein per unit of time rises as the fourth power of the radius (Fig. 32). For example, if a vein with a radius of 1 mm. had a blood flow through it of 10 cc. per minute, an enlargement of the radius to 2 mm., or an increase of only 2 mm. in the diameter, all other factors remaining thesame, would result in a volume of blood flow 16 times greater (2^4) or 160 cc. per minute (Fig. 32). Therefore, the greater the diameter of the lumen of a vein, the greater the volume of blood that flows through it, all other factors remaining unchanged.

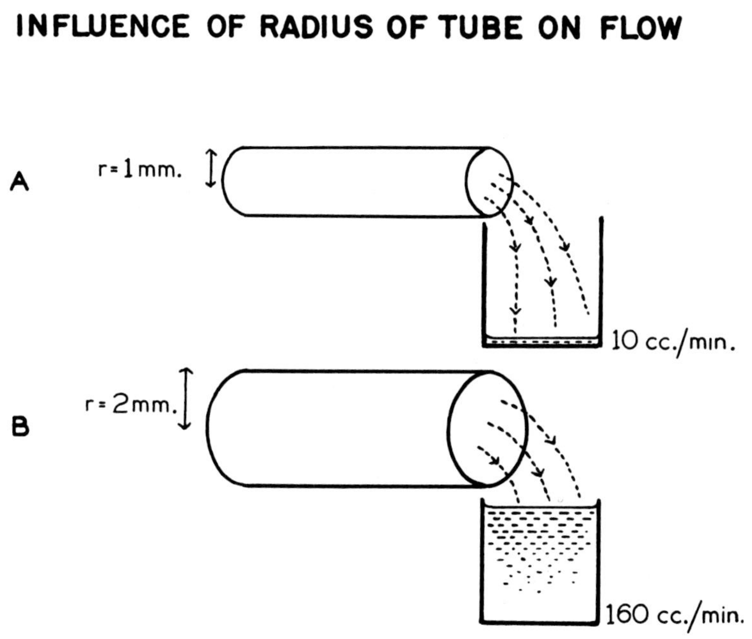

FIG. 32.—The rate of flow of blood through a tube varies directly with the fourth power of the radius. If all factors are constant except the radius and if a vein, *A*, with a radius of 1 mm., has flow of 10 cc. of blood per minute, an increase of the radius to 2 mm., *B*, would increase the blood flow 16 times (2^4).

Pressure Gradient.—Poiseuille's law indicates that the greater the pressure gradient, $\frac{p}{l}$, the greater is the volume flow of blood through a vein, all other factors remaining constant. For example, if a pressure gradient of 5 mm. of water over a segment of vein is increased to 10 mm., the flow is increased by a factor of two or is doubled (Fig. 33). Factors which alter the

INFLUENCE OF PRESSURE GRADIENT IN TUBE ON FLOW

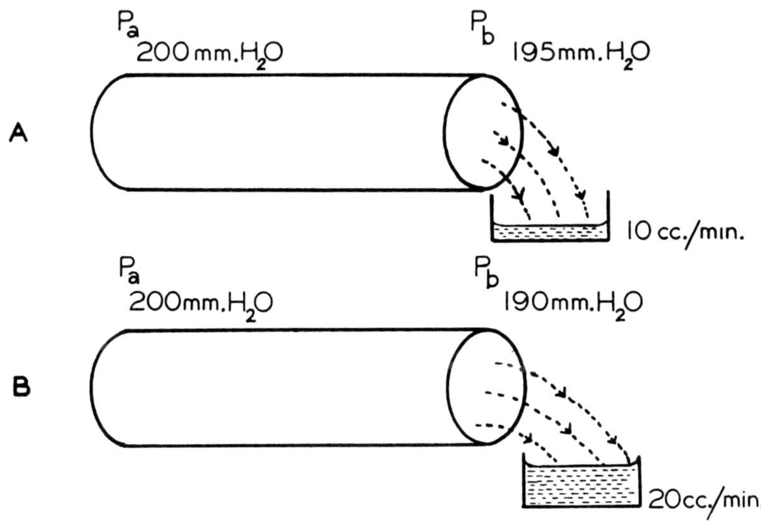

Fig. 33.—The greater the pressure gradient over a given segment of vein, the greater the volume of blood flow through the vein. Venous segment *A* has a pressure head of 5 mm. of water, whereas segment *B* has a pressure head of 10 mm. of water, or twice as large a gradient. Therefore, segment *B* has twice as large a rate of blood flow through it.

pressure gradient in a venous segment will likewise alter directly the rate of volume flow through the vessel. Such variations occur to a great extent in man, as discussed later.

Viscosity of Blood.—The viscosity of the blood flowing through a vein influences the rate of volume flow of blood; the more viscous the blood, the less the flow (Fig. 34). This is well known to everyone from personal experience. For example, oil flows through a given spigot more slowly than water. This inverse relationship is indicated in Poiseuille's equation by the fact that the coefficient of viscosity, η, is in the denominator. Whereas viscosity of the blood remains relatively constant under most circumstances, there are certain special circumstances when it does change. It increases, for example, with hemoconcentration of shock or with polycythemia vera.

INFLUENCE OF VISCOSITY OF FLUID ON FLOW

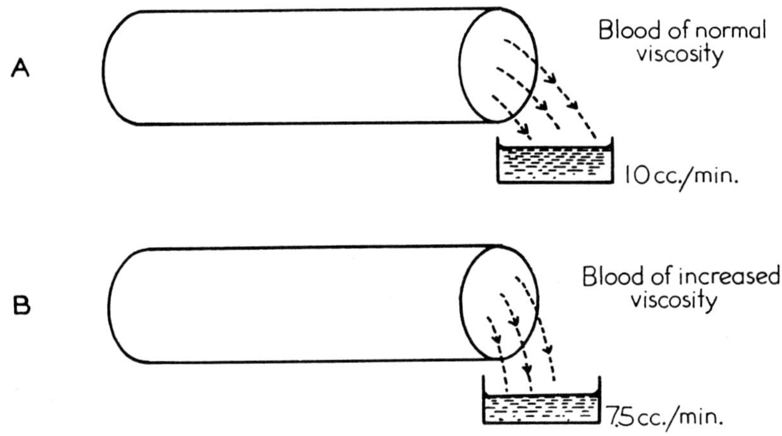

FIG. 34.—An increase in viscosity of blood reduces the rate of blood flow through a vein.

Although any more extensive discussion of Poiseuille's law and its implications is not feasible here, it is well to note that the fall in pressure along a given length of vein can be calculated from the equation:

$$p = \frac{8l\eta v}{980\ r^2} \qquad (3)$$

where p is the fall in pressure in millimeters of water,
l is the length of a segment of vein in millimeters,
v is the mean velocity of flow in millimeters per second, and
r is the radius of the vein in millimeters.

This equation is another variant of Poiseuille's equation discussed previously. Under clinical and most experimental conditions it is more practical to measure the pressure or its changes directly along a segment of vein, but such direct determinations of venous pressure are influenced by many factors which must be properly evaluated. Several of these are noted in equations (2) and (3).

VENOUS PRESSURE

Within a blood vessel, such as a vein, there are two factors which influence recordings of pressure by a direct method:

1) Potential energy, evidenced by lateral pressure
2) Kinetic energy, evidenced by velocity of flow.

1) **Potential Energy and Lateral Pressure.**—A vein becomes distended when pressure acts in a lateral direction upon the internal surfaces of its walls (Fig. 35). Since pressure is force per unit area, for example, pounds

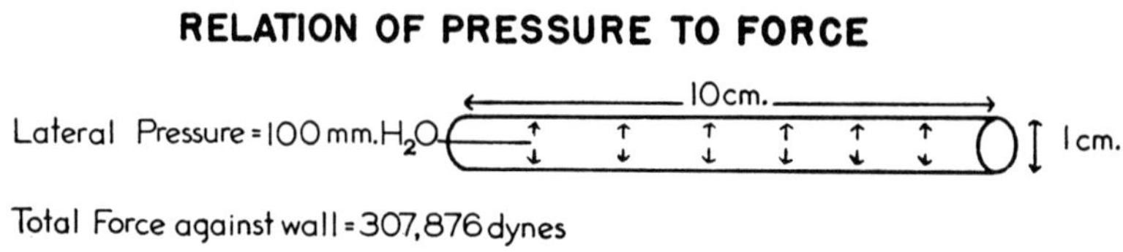

FIG. 35.—Pressure acting laterally upon the internal surfaces of the wall of a vein.

per square inch, atmospheres, or millimeters of water, the total force acting in a lateral direction is expressed by the equation

$$F = PA, \tag{4}$$

where F is force,
P is the pressure, and
A is the total area upon which the pressure is acting.

Thus, for a vessel of the size shown in Figure 35 (surface area of $2\pi rl$ or 31.4 $cm.^2$) and a pressure of 100 mm. of water* the total force acting on the wall would be 307,876 dynes.

The lateral pressure may also be considered to represent the pressure manifested by the *potential energy* within the blood stream. This pressure not only acts laterally but also radially from a point that is also in the direction of, as well as against, the flowing stream of blood (Fig. 36). For

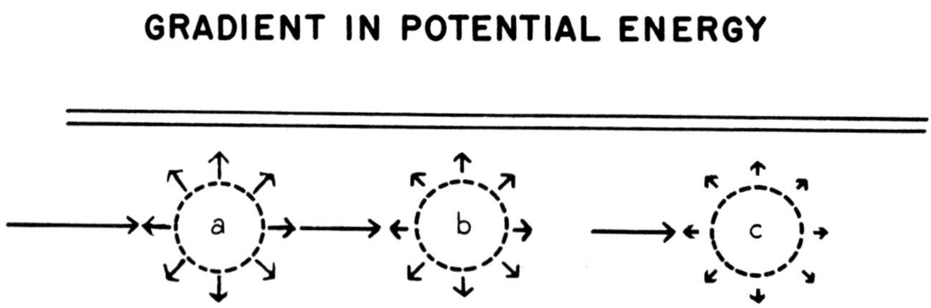

FIG. 36.—Force or pressure, an index of potential energy, acting in all directions radially from three spherical segments within a venous segment with flowing blood. Consult the text for details.

* Ten mm. of water pressure at 4°C. is equal to a force of 980.638 dynes per square centimeter. A dyne is the force that will produce an acceleration of one centimeter per second in a gram mass.

example, if one considers a spherical portion, *a*, within a segment of vein containing flowing blood, it possesses potential energy manifested by pressure acting radially in all directions from the surface of the hypothetic spherical segment. The arrows, which are vector quantities, indicate the magnitude and direction of pressure (Fig. 36). This pressure is counterbalanced by the wall of the vein and the flowing blood, but it remains ready to act or manifest itself as energy at any possible moment. The pressure, an index of available potential energy at any point in a segment of vein, can be measured by means of a tube or needle inserted into the venous segment. Obviously, if blood is flowing from left to right in such a segment, the potential energy and its subsequently manifested pressure or force must be slightly greater in any portion to the left of any other section of the vein, because of loss of energy due to friction. For example, the potential energy in spherical section *b* is less than at section *a* but is greater than that at *c* (Fig. 36). It is important to remember that the energy progressively declines from *a* to *c* because of frictional loss as heat. If potential energies and, therefore, pressures at these three points remained equal, the flow of blood would cease because of friction. If, on the other hand, the potential energy at *c* were greater than that at *b* and if that at *b* were greater than that at *a*, and if the gradient remained as such, then there would be a reversal of flow, *i.e.*, flow would be from right to left. Considerations of kinetic energy must be made, however, and will be discussed later.

Lateral pressure may be measured by the insertion of a tube into a vein with the lumen of the tube directed perpendicular to that of the vein (Fig. 37). Such a tube is known as a Pitot tube, which is the fundamental device employed in measuring venous pressure. Since blood is flowing through the tube and since the plane of the opening in the Pitot tube is parallel to the current of blood flow, true lateral pressure is measured.

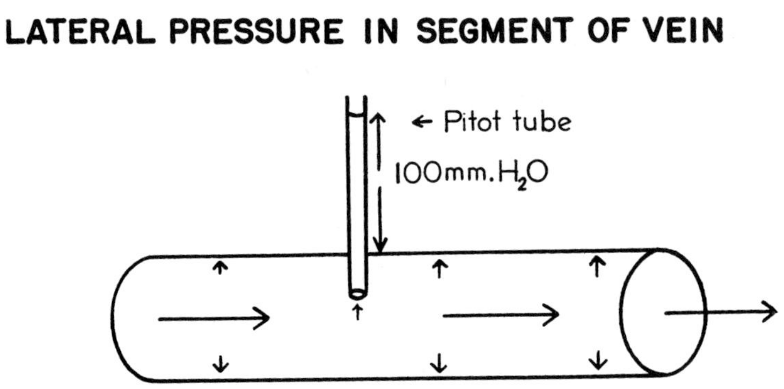

Fig. 37.—Influence of lateral pressure in a segment of vein in maintaining a pressure column of 100 mm. of water.

2) **Pressure Induced by Kinetic Energy.**—A moving mass possesses energy due to its motion. Since this energy of motion, known as kinetic energy (K. E.), is of considerable importance in hemodynamics, especially in vessels in which blood is flowing rapidly, it is advisable to understand its nature.

Consider the kinetic energy of a *unit volume* of blood moving with velocity v at point A (Fig. 38). This unit volume has kinetic energy,

$$\text{K. E.} = \tfrac{1}{2}\,mv^2, \tag{5}$$

where m = mass of the material in grams. However, since unit volume is considered, numerically P = m, where P = density in grams per c.c.; therefore

$$\text{K. E.} = \tfrac{1}{2}\,Pv.^2 \tag{6}$$

Suppose this unit volume of blood strikes the curved vane B, which changes its direction of motion from horizontal to vertical without loss of

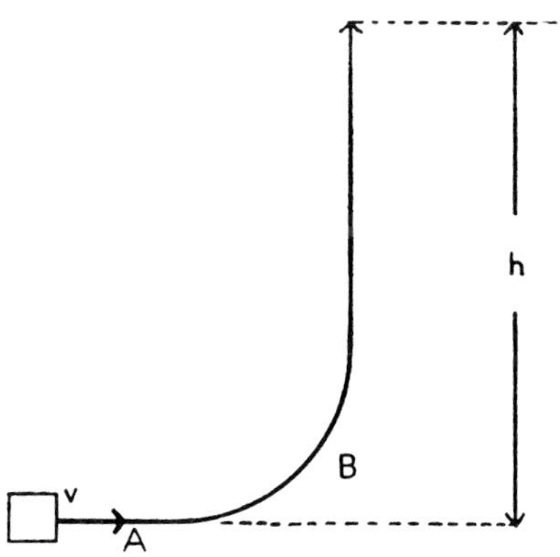

FIG. 38.—Consult the text for details.

energy. As the mass moves upward, its velocity decreases because of gravitational attraction. The velocity will become zero when the mass reaches height h at which its kinetic energy is zero but at which its potential energy (P. E.) as a result of its position is

$$\text{P. E.} = (m \times g) \times h = P \times g \times h, \text{ and} \tag{7}$$

$$\text{P. E.} = \text{K. E., that is} \tag{8}$$

$$\tfrac{1}{2}\,Pv^2 = Pgh \tag{9}$$

$$h = \frac{v^2}{2g}. \tag{10}$$

Therefore, if a Pitot tube is turned to point upstream in a vein transmitting flowing blood, the kinetic energy of the flowing blood will appear on

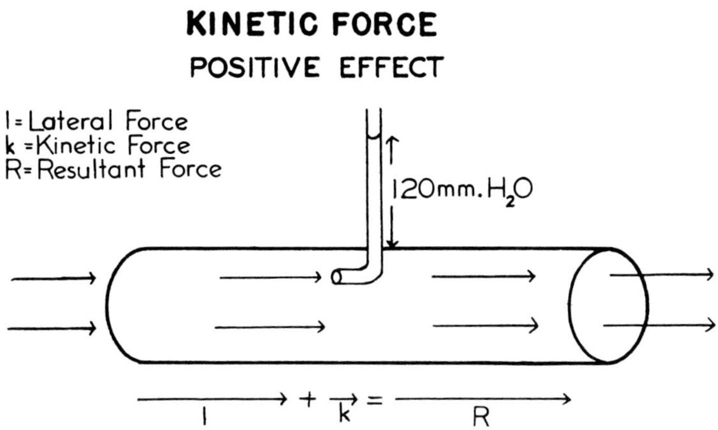

FIG. 39.—A Pitot tube with its orifice directed opposite to or against the flow of blood in a segment of vein. The additive influence of the potential (lateral pressure of 100 mm. of water) and kinetic ("flow" pressure of 20 mm. of water) forces are recorded in the Pitot tube as 120 mm. of water pressure.

the indicator of the Pitot tube as potential energy indicated by an increase in height of blood in the tube by the amount h, where

$$h = \frac{v^2}{2g} \text{ (Fig. 39).}$$

The height to which blood would rise in the Pitot tube would be due to the potential energy manifested by the lateral pressure in the vein plus the kinetic energy which is converted into potential energy as described previously.

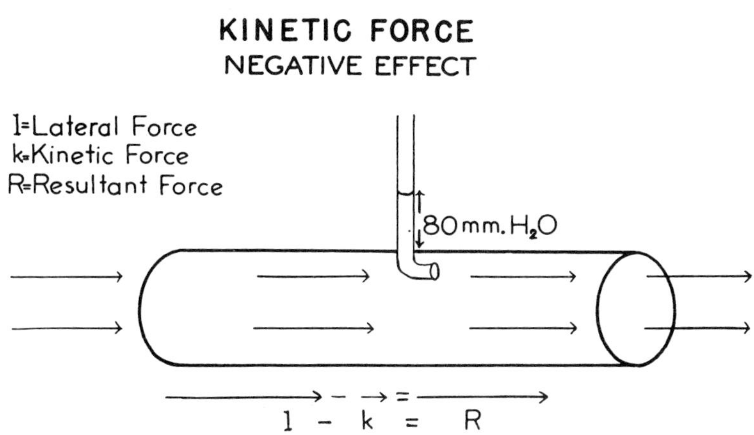

FIG. 40.—A Pitot tube in a vein with flowing blood with its orifice in direction coincident with the direction of blood flow. The recorded pressure is essentially the difference between the potential and kinetic forces, or 80 = 100 − 20 mm. of water.

That a moving stream exerts a force, measurable as pressure, on an obstruction which is proportional to the stream velocity is shown in the case of a stream of water striking a pebble. The pebble is moved in the direction of flow.

If the Pitot tube is pointed downstream, the velocity effect of the fluid is opposite to that in the case of the tube which is pointed upstream. The indicated pressure is less than the static pressure, that is, the pressure recorded would be lateral pressure minus that due to the flowing blood by the amount h (Fig. 40). This effect is shown in an aspiration in which flowing water passing a tube pointed downstream creates a vacuum (negative pressure) in the tube.

A composite picture of the three possible pressure manifestations of potential energy and kinetic energy when a tube is placed in a vein is shown in Figure 41. It is evident, therefore, that the pressure recorded when a

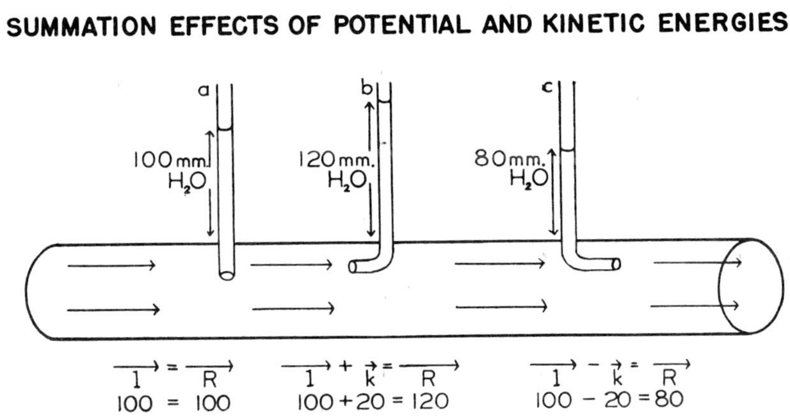

FIG. 41.—Composite illustration showing the effects of potential and kinetic forces on the measured venous pressure. Pitot tube *a* records a true lateral pressure in the venous segment and *b* and *c* the sum of the pressure manifestations of the potential and kinetic forces.

needle is introduced into the flowing blood stream of a vein will depend upon the relation of the direction of the opening of the needle to the direction of blood flow. It is also obvious that the more rapid the blood flow, the greater the influence of the kinetic force. Such phenomena must be borne in mind when measurements of venous pressure are obtained.

Interrelationship of Potential and Kinetic Energies.—It is necessary to consider the interrelationship of the potential and kinetic energies in a segment of vein containing flowing blood, especially under circumstances when one may be converted into the other. This can best be exemplified by blood flowing in an irregularly shaped segment. For example, in a venous segment which has a narrowed portion multiple conversions of potential and kinetic energies will occur in the vicinity of the narrowing (Fig. 42). Figure 42 shows a venous segment containing flowing blood in which a portion of its lumen is constricted. At a distance from the constricted portion the energy possessed by the flowing blood is divided into potential and kinetic, the former being greater. In this illustration, neglecting energy loss by friction, the potential energy is indicated by its manifestation as lateral pressure,

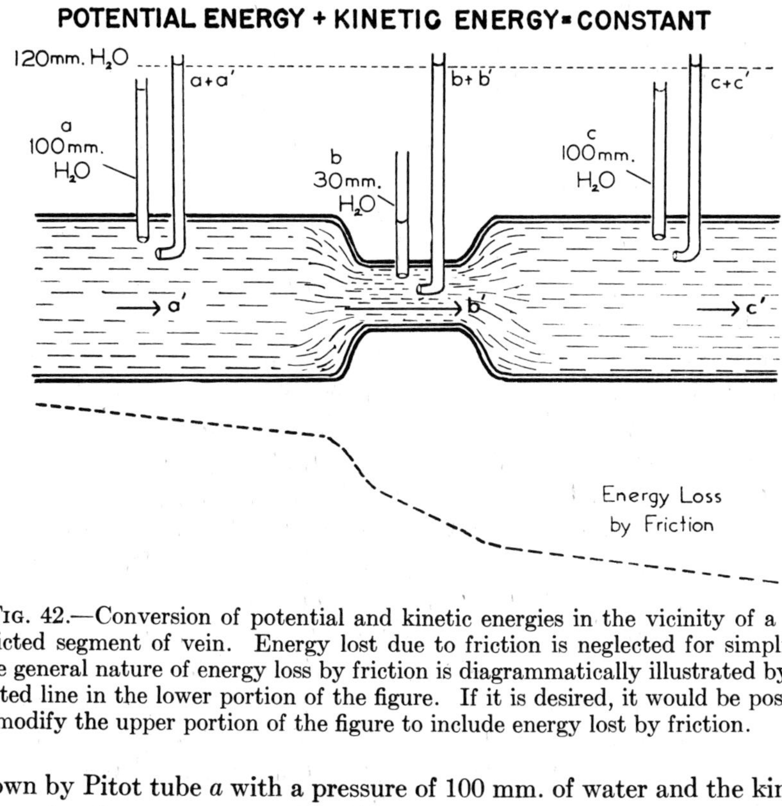

FIG. 42.—Conversion of potential and kinetic energies in the vicinity of a constricted segment of vein. Energy lost due to friction is neglected for simplicity The general nature of energy loss by friction is diagrammatically illustrated by the dotted line in the lower portion of the figure. If it is desired, it would be possible to modify the upper portion of the figure to include energy lost by friction.

shown by Pitot tube *a* with a pressure of 100 mm. of water and the kinetic energy by the vector *a′* capable of offering a pressure of 20 mm. of water. The total energy, therefore, develops a pressure of 120 mm. of water.

Obviously, the amount of blood flowing per unit of time through the section of the vein in the vicinity of Pitot tubes *a*, *b* and *c* or through any cross section of venous segment shown in Figure 42 must be equal. Therefore, since the diameter of the lumen in the constricted portion is considerably less than that in any other portion, the linear rate of blood flow there must be greater than in the nonconstricted portions. Therefore, except for the loss in energy due to friction, the sum of the potential and kinetic energies in the constricted portion must equal the sum of those in the nonconstricted portions; the magnitude of the kinetic energy in the constricted portion increases (capable of exerting a pressure of 90 mm. of water), vector *b′*, and the potential energy manifested by the lateral pressure *b* (30 mm. of water) decreases proportionately. Potential energy is thus converted into kinetic energy, the total energy remaining the same, as indicated by a total pressure of 120 mm. being developed by the two types of energy.

When the blood passes from the narrow, constricted segment into the wider, nonconstricted portion, the velocity of flow decreases and kinetic energy is reconverted into potential energy, or vector *c′* becomes smaller than vector *b′* and likewise the manifested lateral pressure in Pitot tube *c* is greater than that in tube *b*. Then as blood flow becomes restabilized, as indicated by the Pitot tube *c*, the kinetic energy, vector *c′*, is the same as *a′*, since the linear rates of flow and volume rates of flow are equivalent in these two regions. The potential energy manifested by the lateral pressure of 100 mm. of water recorded by Pitot tube *c* would be less than that at Pitot tube *a* if the frictional loss of energy as heat occurring in the vicinity of the constriction had not been ignored.

Of course, there is energy loss due to friction in a tube containing flowing fluid, as shown in Figure 42. The loss in energy in the segment is diagrammatically shown by the dotted line near the lower portion of the illustration. The energy is lost as heat and is never regained. Since the total pressure that may be developed at a given point in the system is dependent upon the total energy present at that point, this dotted line also indicates the change in total pressure along the segment that would occur had frictional loss of energy been considered in the foregoing discussion.

Therefore, according to *Bernoulli's theorem*, at any point in a tube through which a liquid is flowing the sum of the potential energy, positional energy and kinetic energy, is constant. This sum would also be constant for any point along a segment of a tube if frictional loss of energy did not occur. However, as Poiseuille's law indicates, there is frictional loss of energy due to viscosity of the flowing fluid.

Bernoulli's law for any point in a tube may be expressed by the equation:

$$P + hdg + \tfrac{1}{2}\, dv^2 = K, \qquad (11)$$

where P is pressure,
h is the height above a reference plane,
d is the density of the liquid,
g is gravity,
v is the velocity of flow, and
K is a constant.

This theorem has many physiologic applications and is important in the finer applications of venous pressure to clinical problems, but most of the important applications are self-evident and will be discussed only briefly. Aspects of this have been discussed previously with the presentation of the nature of kinetic energy and its conversion to potential energy (pages 44, 47).

If the constricted lumen were extremely narrow and the linear rate of blood flow were rapid, the lateral pressure may become negative, or some of the potential energy of the tissues and atmosphere outside of the vein might even be converted into kinetic energy of flow within the vein. The water suction pump so commonly employed in laboratories makes use of these principles.

The foregoing discussions and illustrations demonstrate the manner in which venous pressure varies in a venous segment containing a constricted portion. The greater the velocity of the blood in a venous segment, the greater will be the conversion phenomena and therefore the greater the variations in lateral pressure. Such variations are likely to be encountered in the head and neck or the elevated arm. Such factors must be considered for proper evaluations of venous pressure. It is also possible to understand from Figure 42 the manner in which venous hums may develop near constricted or distorted portions of venous lumina. These local disturbances in hemodynamics occur at local areas of vasoconstriction, around improperly functioning or diseased venous valves, areas of extrinsic pressure, and kinks.

INFLUENCE OF THE SHAPE OF VEINS ON HEMODYNAMICS

The shape of the veins influences the hemodynamic state within them. A vein which is fully distended allows a larger volume of flow, all other factors remaining constant, than one partially collapsed, because the friction per unit volume of flow is greater in the latter. A larger proportion of the

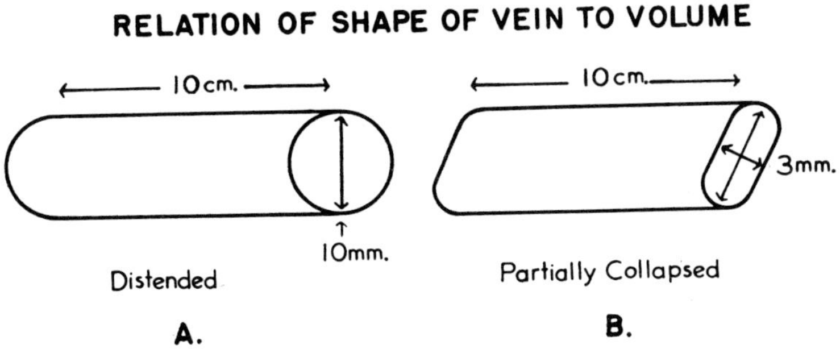

FIG. 43.—The segment of vein *A* would have less surface area per unit volume of blood than segment *B*. Per unit volume of fluid flowing through segments *A* and *B*, there would be more loss of energy due to friction in segment *B* than in segment *A*.

volume of blood is in contact with the surface of the partially collapsed vein than with that of a distended one (Fig. 43). This relatively larger surface area in contact with the flowing blood produces a larger amount of friction or resistance to flow per unit volume of blood (Fig. 44).

Variations in venous configuration influence resistance to blood flow, which in turn tends to maintain a constant pressure in certain veins even when position is suddenly changed. For example, when a man suddenly sits erect from the supine position, blood tends to drain suddenly out of the cerebral veins. However, sudden emptying of the cerebral veins is inhibited, partly because the jugular veins in the neck collapse, so that resistance to flow is increased, and obstruction to venous flow tends to occur (Fig. 45). Furthermore, the pressure in these vital veins is maintained, and the hemodynamic state in the cerebral vessels is not altered unduly.

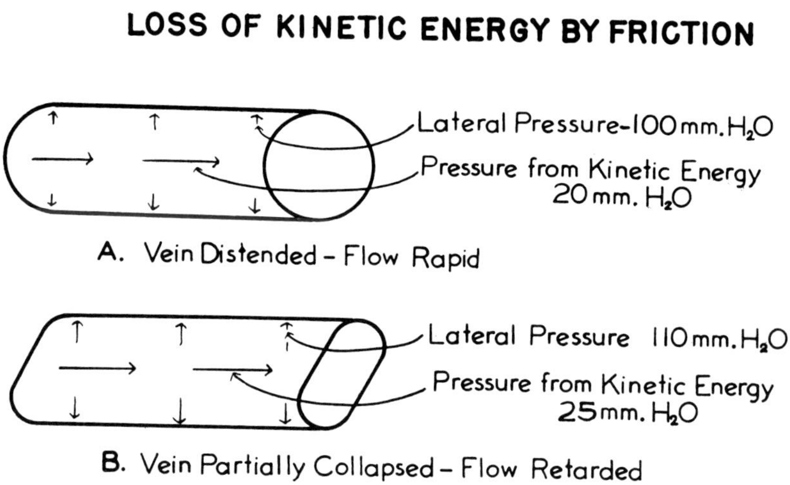

FIG. 44.—To insure an equal flow, the energy necessary to maintain this flow would have to be greater in segment *B* than in segment *A* because of greater loss of energy due to friction. Therefore, the pressures manifested by potential energy and kinetic energy would be greater in *B* than in *A*. If the source of energy remained unchanged, the rate of volume flow through tube *A* would be greater than through tube B and the potential and kinetic energies would be less in *B* than in *A*.

It is interesting to note that the cerebral sinusoids tend to maintain their pressure even when the position of the body is varied. Because they are not collapsible, blood cannot rush out of the sinusoids when a person suddenly sits erect. If they could collapse suddenly like the jugular vein, they would empty as rapidly as the veins of the neck. The volume of blood within them remains practically unchanged when the sitting position is assumed. The same hemodynamic phenomenon applies to the venous sinusoids of the liver, bones, and spleen, which do not collapse readily or at all. Therefore, the pressure within these venous sinusoids tends to remain essentially uniform, and these vital organs tend to maintain uniform circulation and essentially stable hemodynamic state, which are so important for healthy function and metabolism.

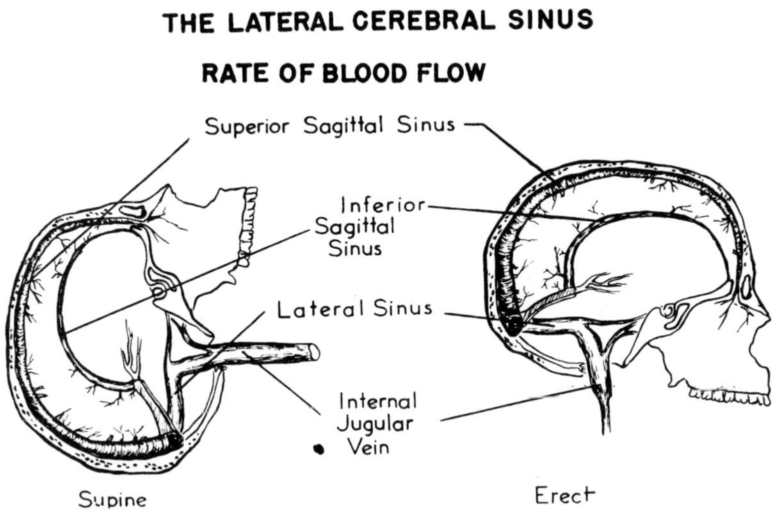

FIG. 45.—When the subject is in the supine position, the jugular vein is distended; when he is in the sitting position, this vein is collapsed, which tends to inhibit venous flow from cerebral sinusoids.

PRESSURE GRADIENT IN THE VENOUS SYSTEM

The pressure is highest in the aorta and declines as the arterioles and capillaries are approached. The pressure, as it is usually recorded, is a manifestion of potential and kinetic energies described previously for the veins. The lumina of the individual arterial vessels are large centrally, decreasing progressively as the periphery is approached. Since the lumina of the vessels decrease in diameter and increase in number, a greater pressure head is required to force the blood peripherally due to greater surface area and frictional resistance (Fig. 46). *Because of the heart,* a considerable pressure head can be developed which will force blood through the arterial and arteriolar systems of tubes. The pressure decreases on the arterial side from the heart to the periphery.

The situation in the venous system of vessels is different from that on the arterial side. The pressure declines from the capillaries to the heart, being positive in the capillaries and venules and approximately zero in the vena cavae near the heart. The level of pressure in the venules is not high nor is

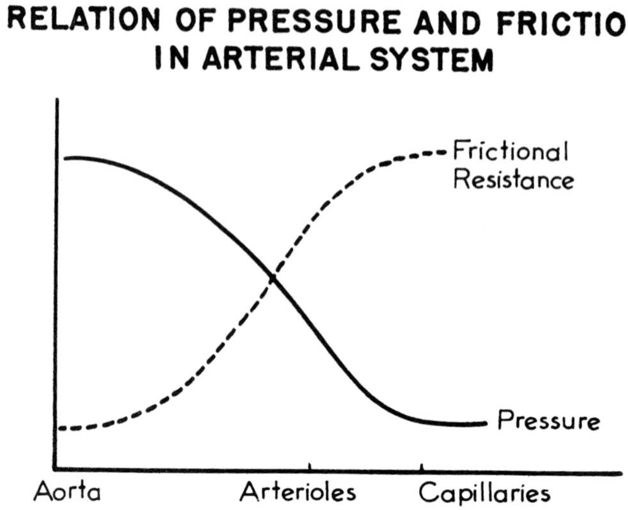

FIG. 46.—Variations in pressure and friction in the arterial side of the circulatory system.

the absolute magnitude of its variations as great as on the arterial side, except perhaps on a percentage basis. However, on the venous side of the circulation the amount of frictional resistance decreases as the heart is approached (Fig. 47). Therefore, although there is a decline in pressure level, there is also a decrease in the pressure gradient and absolute energy required to maintain flow. The number of small vessels decreases and the

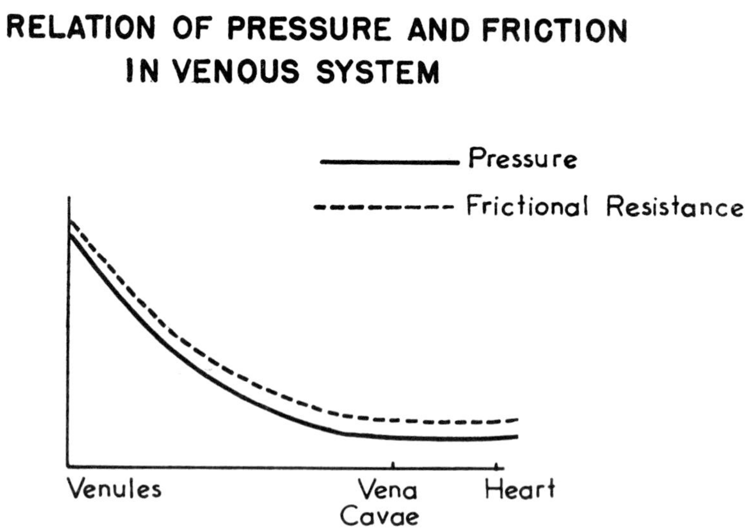

FIG. 47.—Variations in pressure and friction in the venous side of the circulatory system.

frictional area decreases; therefore, the rate of energy dissipation per unit distance or decline in pressure gradient tends to be reduced as the heart is approached.

It is possible to visualize the arterial side of the circulation as a high pressure system with a narrow stopcock at the exit (Fig. 48). This stopcock is represented by the arterioles which reduce the pressure of the blood before it enters the capillaries by offering frictional resistance to blood flow. The

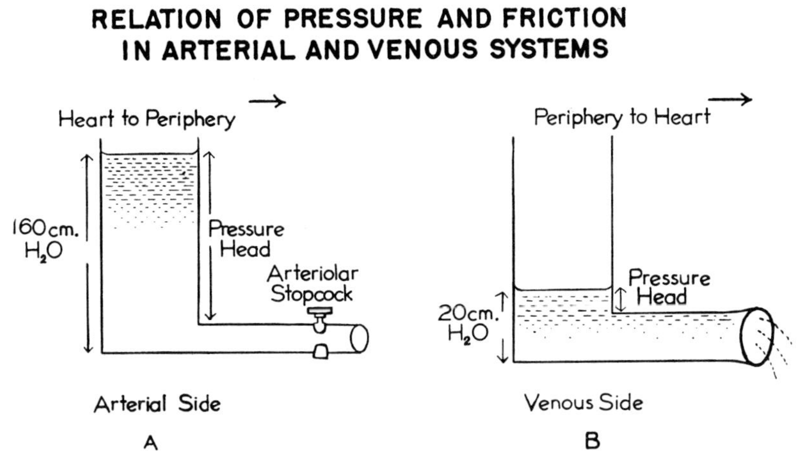

FIG. 48.—*A*, Arterial side with large pressure head has system of "stopcocks" (arterioles) in periphery, which offer resistance to intra-arterial pressure. *B*, Venous side of circulation has small pressure head but no "stopcocks" to obstruct flow; in fact, low intrathoracic pressure and ever-enlarging vessels from periphery to heart facilitate flow.

venous side of the circulation with its low pressure head but ever-increasing size of the blood vessels as the heart is approached, low intrathoracic pressure, and ever-decreasing frictional resistance from periphery to the heart, makes the relatively low pressure head effective in insuring a rate of return flow to the heart equal to the rate of outflow from the heart maintained by the larger arterial pressure head.

FACTORS FAVORING VENOUS RETURN TO THE HEART AND A VENOUS PRESSURE GRADIENT

As stated previously, in order for the blood to flow through the veins from the tissues to the heart it is necessary that a pressure gradient be maintained most of the time, with the higher level of pressure in the venules and the lower level in the vena cavae at the right atrium. Measurements of venous pressure in normal man have shown this gradient to exist and those which fail to reveal such a gradient are in error or indicate disease. Therefore, any values of venous pressure which indicate a higher pressure in a segment of vein more centrally located than in an adjoining more peripheral portion are either evidence of a physiologic disturbance or of an error in measurement.

For a better appreciation of the clinical importance of this gradient it is necessary to have a knowledge of the factors concerned with the return of blood from the tissues to the heart. Only general factors are considered here, though there are many special circumstances or situations, such as portal venous flow through the liver, which are not clearly understood and which are too specialized to warrant a detailed discussion. Among the factors affecting and usually aiding venous return are:

1) Force or pressure originating in the heart, "*vis a tergo*"
2) Negative intrathoracic pressure
3) Function of right ventricle
4) Contraction of noncardiac muscle
5) Gravity
6) Relative volume of blood in arterial and venous systems
7) Venous tone.

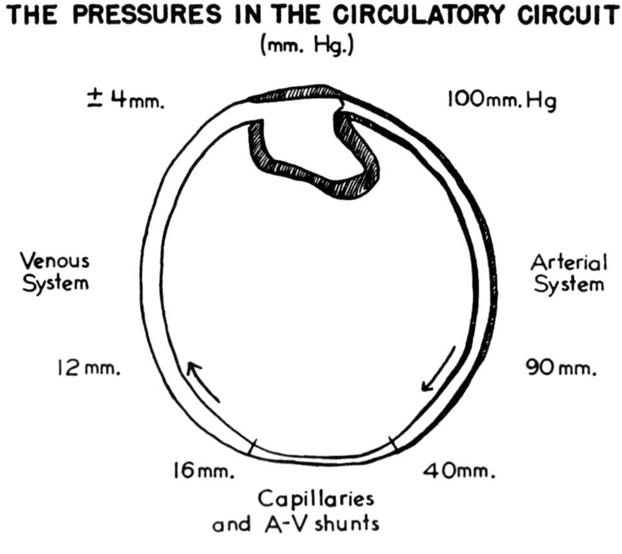

FIG. 49.—The circulation is a continuous system of open tubes; therefore, pressure developed in the heart might be expected to be transmitted into the venous side. Numerals indicate approximate values of pressure in millimeters of mercury within various portions of the normal active circulation. The gradient is from the left side to the right side of the heart.

1) **Force of Cardiac Systole.**—Since the circulation is a continuous circuit of tubes and the heart is a pump which is responsible for establishing a pressure head, the pressure, manifestations of potential and kinetic energies, developed by the heart might be expected to be conducted and to penetrate throughout this open circuit of tubes (Fig. 49). The gradient in pressure is from the left ventricle to the right atrium, the highest pressure being in the aorta and the lowest in the vena cavae at their entrance into the right atrium. The most rapid rate of decline in pressure occurs in the arteriolar portions of the circulation (Fig. 50). The arterioles act as stopcocks which intervene between the arterial and venous sides of the circulation (Fig. 51). The

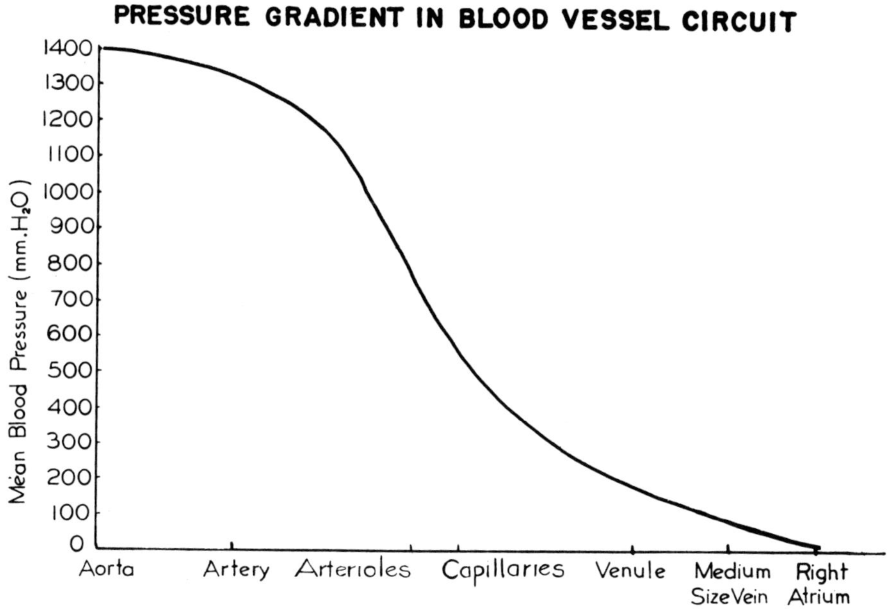

FIG. 50.—Diagram of the pressure gradient of the circulatory system. (Modified from Landis, Physiol. Rev., *14*, 416, 1934).

tighter the stopcocks are closed, *i. e.*, the greater the arteriolar constriction, the greater the drop in pressure or the less the pressure or force or energy which is transmitted into the venous side of the circulation (Fig. 51). If the arteriolar constriction were sufficiently great to occlude the arteriolar lumen completely, circulation would cease and no pressure would be transmitted to the venous side of the circulation (Fig. 51 *A*). The pressure in the arterial side of the system would become equalized at a pressure below systolic if cardiac action also were temporarily stopped. Therefore, no pressure could be transmitted from the arterial side of the circulation into the venous side, and the influence of the *vis a tergo* would be eliminated. The pressure in the venous system would tend to decline but would not reach zero because of tone of the muscles and walls of the veins and tissue pressure.

When the arterioles are partially constricted, a continuous lumen is maintained between the arterial and venous systems, and pressure from the arterial side can be transmitted to the venous system (Fig. 51 *B*). This is essentially the condition existing in normal resting man. The pressure transmitted from the arterial side is available to force blood back to the heart, and a continually beating heart maintains this *vis a tergo*.

Under certain circumstances the arterioles may become greatly dilated so that the "stopcocks" enlarge the lumen connecting the arterial and venous sides of the circulation. This facilitates transmission of force, or potential and kinetic energies, from the arterial side and thereby increases

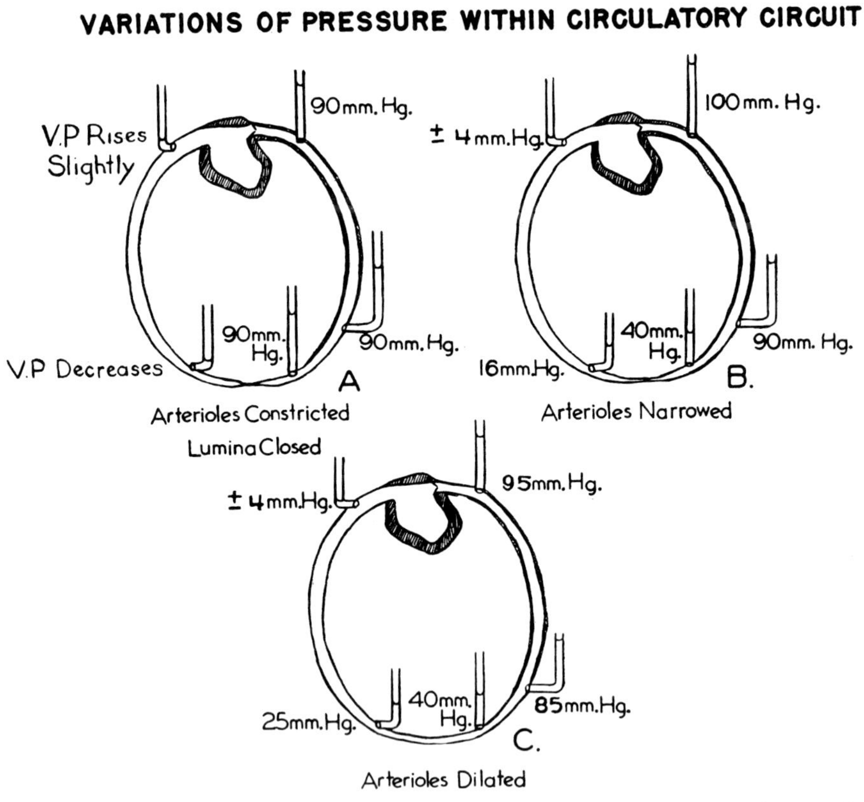

FIG. 51.—Transmission of pressure or, more correctly, energy from the arteria side of the circulation. The arterioles behave as "stopcocks," the degree with which they are constricted or dilated determines distribution and magnitude of pressure within the circulatory system. *A* shows the arterioles closed for a short moment with cardiac asystole, *B* and *C* show an active circulation and are self-explanatory. The pressure values are not necessarily average normal.

the pressure head forcing blood back to the heart through the venous system (Fig. 51 *C*). Under such circumstances the absolute values of the venous and, of course, arterial pressures would be altered.

Included in the arteriolar portion of the circulation are the various types of direct arteriovenous anastomoses (Fig. 52), which permit more direct transmission of energy or pressure from the arterial to the venous system. Since their lumina are usually larger and fewer in number, they offer less frictional resistance to flow than the capillaries. A large *vis a tergo* is thus made available to force blood into the venous system toward the heart. Because of their number, these shunts are important in maintaining venous pressure and venous flow.

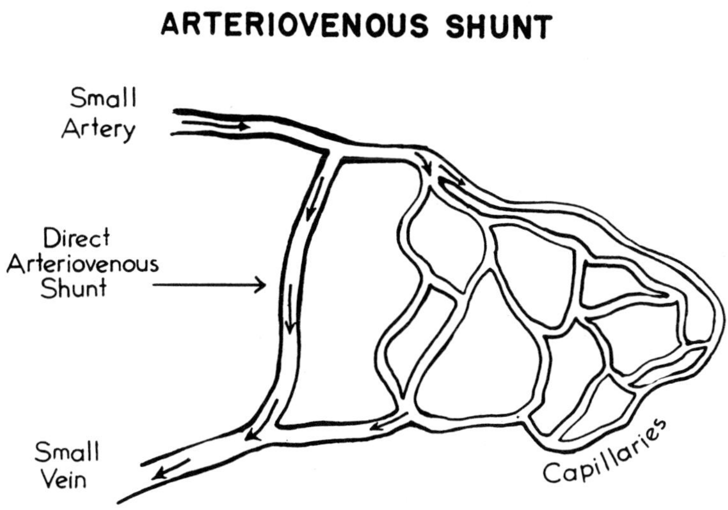

FIG. 52.—Direct arteriovenous shunt which permits better transmission of energy or pressure from arterial to venous system.

A special application of arteriovenous shunt which is concerned with maintaining venous pressure is that in the portal venous system. The portal vein and its tributaries obtain much of their pressure head from such shunts in the numerous villi of the gastrointestinal tract (Fig. 53). The blood is shunted through a short direct arteriovenous anastomotic vessel and arterial pressure is transmitted directly into the venous side of the circulation to provide *vis a tergo,* so important in supplying a pressure head for the portal venous system. In this way, energy is not lost, as it would be if the blood had circulated through the small capillaries with their high frictional resistance to flow. Energy lost in the capillaries by friction is wasted as far as *vis a tergo* is concerned.

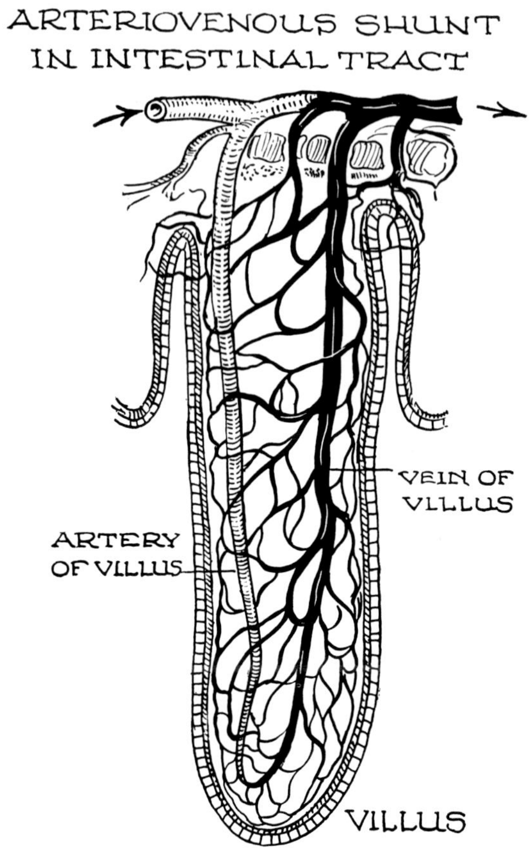

Fig. 53.—Arteriovenous shunt in a villus of the jejunum.

2) **Negative Intrathoracic Pressure.**—During respiration intrathoracic pressure varies, rising above atmospheric pressure with expiration and declining to a level below atmospheric pressure with inspiration. These variations in pressure provide a "pumping" action. The negative or subatmospheric pressure is transmitted into the veins, reducing the venous pressure in the intrathoracic portion of the vena cavae (Fig. 54). This decreases resistance to flow, potential energy or lateral pressure locally and has, according to usual concepts, a "suction" effect on the veins. Reduction of the pressure within the veins to subatmospheric level assists in venous flow toward the heart. This "pumping action" of the thorax is important in venous blood flow. Furthermore, the pressure in the large veins near the thorax will show variations with respiration, a fall with inspiration and a rise with expiration. The importance of these respiratory effects on venous return is best emphasized by the influences of emphysema upon venous return. Emphysema, because of its tendency to

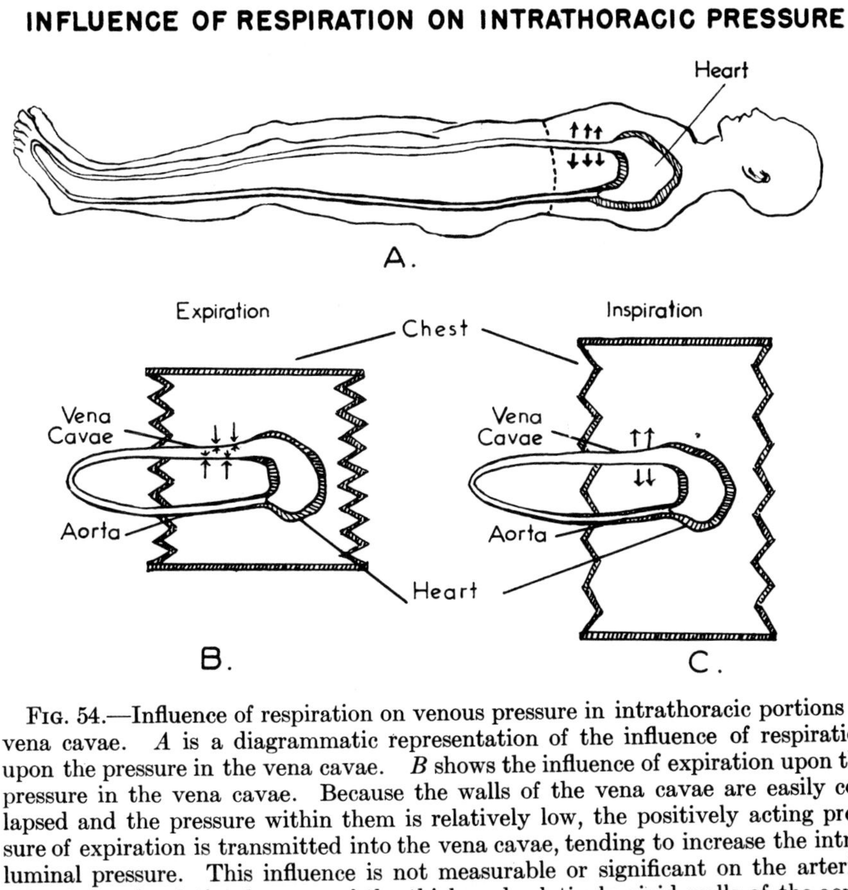

FIG. 54.—Influence of respiration on venous pressure in intrathoracic portions of vena cavae. *A* is a diagrammatic representation of the influence of respiration upon the pressure in the vena cavae. *B* shows the influence of expiration upon the pressure in the vena cavae. Because the walls of the vena cavae are easily collapsed and the pressure within them is relatively low, the positively acting pressure of expiration is transmitted into the vena cavae, tending to increase the intraluminal pressure. This influence is not measurable or significant on the arterial side of the circulation because of the thick and relatively rigid walls of the aorta and arteries and because of the high arterial pressure. *C* shows the influence of inspiration upon the pressure within the vena cava, tending to decrease the pressure. *It is obvious that the "effective" venous pressure, as far as venous return to the heart is concerned, cannot be determined from the venous pressure alone but is rather determined from a proper integration of venous pressure and intrathoracic pressure.*

increase the level of intrathoracic pressure, tends to inhibit venous return and at least reduces or eliminates the respiratory pumping action, and venous pressure tends to be increased in this condition (Fig. 55). This is discussed in greater detail later.

The veins in the chest are easily influenced by the intrathoracic pressure because of their thin pliable walls and the relatively low pressure within these vessels. Variations in extravenous pressure are transmitted into the

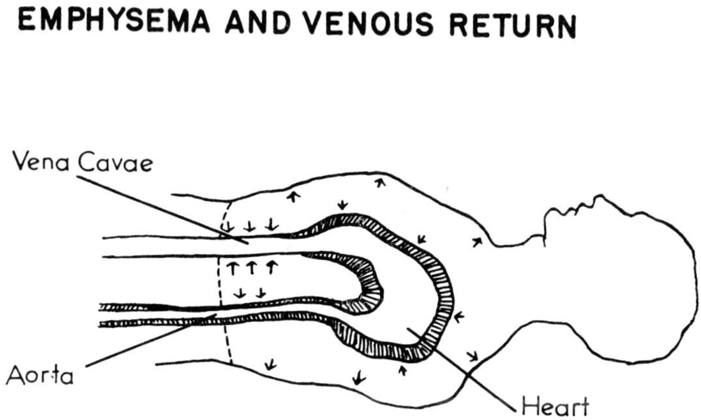

FIG. 55.—The higher intrathoracic pressure in emphysema increases venous pressure in the vena cavae by reducing the "effective" pressure in the vena cavae, *i. e.*, the difference between venous pressure and intrathoracic pressure is decreased. This tends to impair venous return to the heart.

lumen and contents of veins. Being rigid, the arterial walls, including the aorta, are little influenced by the relatively small variations in intrathoracic or extra-arterial pressure.

As indicated previously, not only are the walls of veins soft and pliable but, in addition, the pressure within them is relatively low, so that variations in extravenous pressure, as the intrathoracic pressure, will produce considerable change in venous pressure (Fig. 56). On the other hand, arterial pressure is relatively high, so that even if variations in intrathoracic pressure did affect intra-arterial pressure, the percentage change would be negligible (Fig. 56).

It should be remembered that although respiration tends to influence the vessels of both the superior and inferior vena cavae, the phases of respiration have opposite effects on portions of them. For example, during *inspiration* intra-abdominal pressure is increased as the diaphragm descends. This increases the venous pressure in the intra-abdominal portion of the inferior vena cava and all its tributaries. Simultaneously the venous pressure is reduced in the entire superior vena cava and all its tributaries.

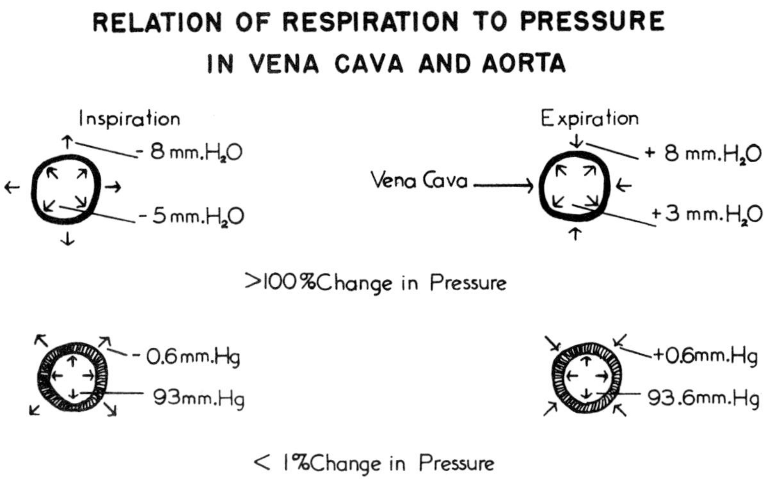

FIG. 56.—Relative change in pressure in the vena cava and aorta produced by phases of respiration. A large percentage change occurs within the vena cava and small change in the aorta even if all effects of intrathoracic pressure are considered to be transmitted into the aorta. Thus the "effective" venous pressure is influenced considerably by respiration but the "effective" arterial pressure is not.

This favors venous return from the superior vena cava and its tributaries and tends to impair return from the tributaries of the intra-abdominal portion of the inferior vena cava. Venous pressure, however, is reduced simultaneously during inspiration in all veins of those portions of both the superior and inferior vena cavae found within the thorax. *Expiration*, on the other hand, increases the pressure in the intrathoracic veins and the tributaries of the superior vena cava, impairing venous return from the head, neck, and arms. As the diaphragm ascends with expiration, intra-abdominal pressure declines, as does the pressure within the intra-abdominal veins, favoring blood flow into them from the extra-abdominal tributaries. Thus, breathing produces phasic increases in venous return toward the heart. The relationship of venous pressure to intrathoracic and intra-abdominal pressure is important in determining venous return (Fig. 57).

3) **Function of the Right Ventricle.**—The right ventricle plays an important role in maintenance of the normal pressure gradient in the veins. If it did not pass on the blood delivered to the right side of the heart, blood would accumulate. The pressure in the veins would increase very slightly, however, because of the great distensibility of the veins and relatively small volume of blood normally present in the pulmonary vessels (Fig. 58). As blood accumulates, the return to the left ventricle is reduced, thereby reducing the output of that ventricle to that of the right ventricle. A new steady state is achieved with each ventricle expelling a reduced but equal

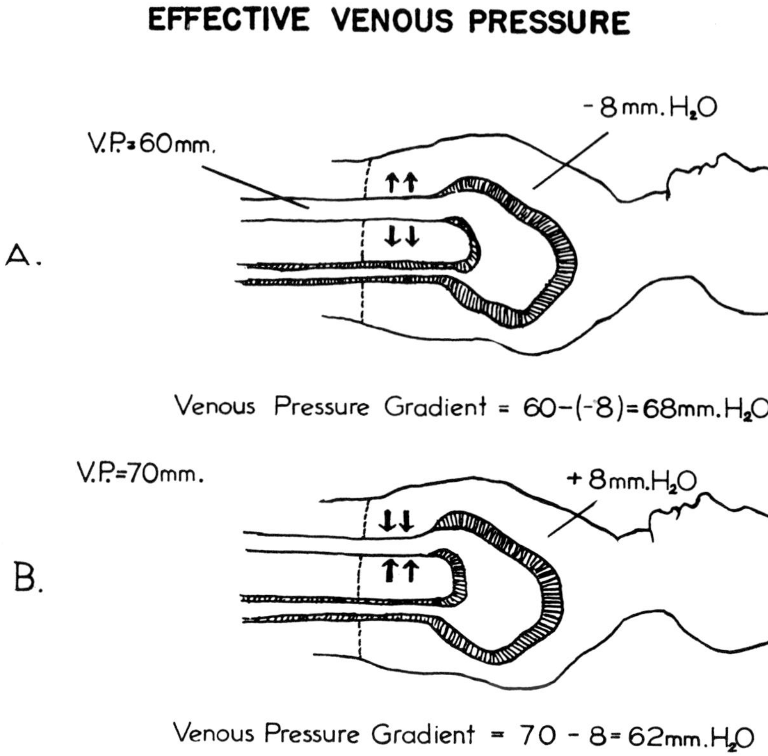

FIG. 57.—Influence of intrathoracic pressure on "effective" venous pressure. It is the difference between the venous pressure and intrathoracic pressure that determines the "effective" venous pressure, or the pressure which is actually concerned with effecting venous return of blood to the heart. For example, the venous pressure is lower for the circumstances shown in *A* than in *B*, but the effective pressure is larger in *A* and venous return would be larger than in *B*.

volume of blood. Unless blood volume is increased or the tone of the vascular system is increased, venous pressure will return to essentially normal levels. It is only with the introduction of other factors, such as reduced urinary volume or the shift of fluid from the intra- and intercellular spaces or both, that blood volume can be increased. The role of humoral or neurogenic factors in influencing blood volume and vascular tone remains vague. Nevertheless, it is important to realize that the failure of the right ventricle to pump blood forward without an associated change in vascular tone, at least venous, or blood volume or both, venous pressure can show only a slight and only a temporary rise.

Although it is stated by many observers that there is no evidence to support the concept that the right ventricle "sucks" blood into it as a syringe or rubber bulb "sucks" up water, there are experiments, for example those of Wiggers, which show the pressure within the ventricles to be declining while they are filling with blood during the diastolic phase. This could only occur with a "suction" effect from the ventricles. A negative pressure has not been noted in the right ventricle during diastole, however. This is not necessary, since it is pressure differential which is important in determining whether or not there is suction.

RIGHT VENTRICULAR FAILURE AND VENOUS INFLOW

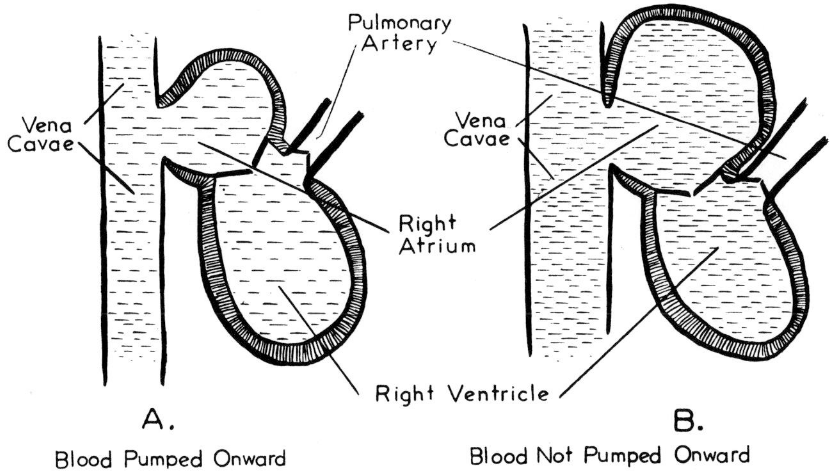

FIG. 58.—*A*, Right ventricle is able to pump blood onward that is delivered to it. Blood does not accumulate in the vena cavæ, and venous pressure is maintained at the normal level. *B*, Right ventricle is not able to pump blood effectively. Blood accumulates in the right atrium and vena cavæ, and the venous pressure increases slightly. These structures become engorged with blood and dilate. This is only temporary. See text.

Therefore, it is important to remember that adequate "passing on" of blood delivered to the right ventricle by the venous system is necessary for proper venous flow, as well as for maintenance of a normal pressure gradient or normal venous pressure throughout the venous system. Disease states which affect the right ventricle might alter the pumping function and bring about decompensation. This results in accumulation of blood in the venous system and accompanying venous hypertension.

4) **Contraction of Noncardiac Muscle.**—The pumping action of the skeletal muscles in assisting venous return has been discussed (page 26). Because of the venous valves it is possible for contraction of skeletal muscles to behave as venous pumps. When a skeletal muscle like the gastrocnemius contracts, intramuscular pressure rises to levels above that in the veins coursing through the muscle (Fig. 59). During the relaxed state of the muscle, when the pressure of the muscular tissue is lower than the pressure of the blood within the veins coursing through the muscle, the veins are able to distend and become filled with blood (Fig. 59 *A*). Blood flows out of the intramuscular veins when the pressure within them exceeds that in the large collecting veins outside the muscle. When the muscle contracts, the pressure of the muscular tissue rises above that within the veins of the muscle, forcibly squeezing the veins and emptying their contents into the large collecting veins outside the muscle (Fig. 59 *B*). When the muscle relaxes again, pressure of the muscular tissue falls below the pressure within the veins of the muscle. Blood suddenly tends to flow back from the large collecting veins outside the muscle to refill the intramuscular veins.

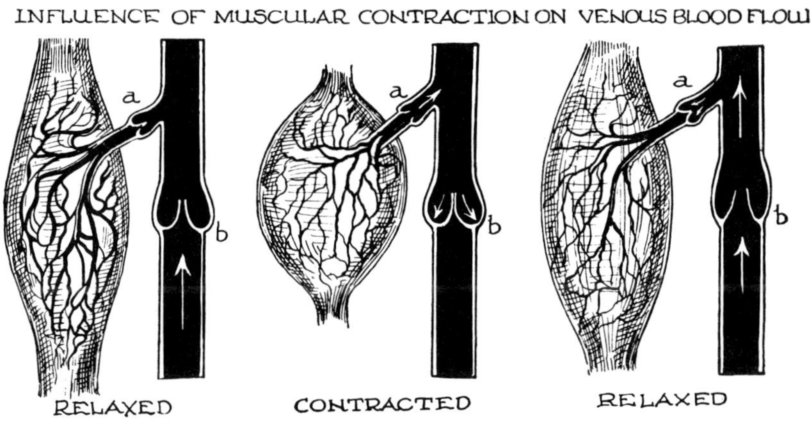

FIG. 59.—Effect of musclar contraction on venous flow.

This reversal of flow is stopped, however, by valves located in the veins at their exit from the muscle. Therefore, the blood squeezed or pumped out of the muscle when it contracts must flow toward the heart. During muscular relaxation the veins within the muscles refill with blood delivered to them from the arterial side of the circulation.

During vigorous exercise involving all the muscles of the body a considerable quantity of blood is "pumped" toward the heart under a fairly high pressure head. This results in an efficient venous flow necessary to meet the demands of rapid metabolism and fairly frequent re-use of the relatively fixed blood volume to meet the requirements of any emergency. Under such circumstances of muscular contraction the venous pressure varies as indicated in Chapter 4.

5) **Gravity.**—The force of gravity has considerable effect upon venous circulation, but the influence varies from time to time. For example, when a man is lying in bed the forces of gravity are exerting minimum influence upon the circulation. When he stands, however, the gravitational force has its greatest effect (Fig. 60), for it assists venous return of blood from the upper portions of the body and impairs return from the lower portions. This force produces a pressure head equal to a column of blood of a length equal to the distance from the vein under consideration to the level of the heart or the phlebostatic level (Fig. 60 *B*). The full gravitational force, however, is not able to manifest itself in the upper portions of the body such as the head because the veins of the neck collapse and, therefore, increase frictional losses of pressure.

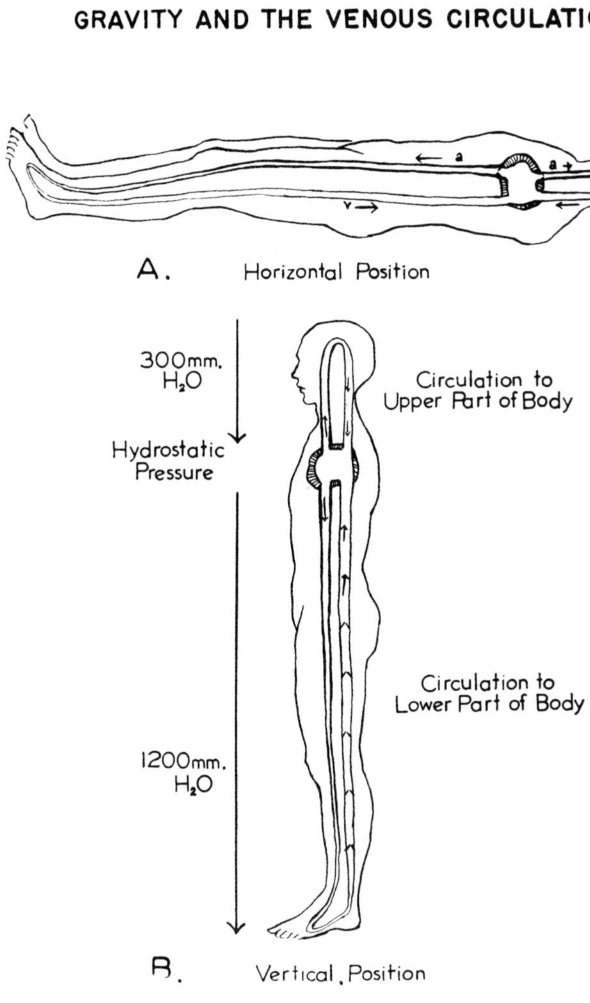

Fig. 60.—Influence of gravity upon venous circulation in lying and standing positions. Large dark arrows are vectors indicating direction and magnitude of force of gravity.

In a man in the standing position the force of gravity inhibits venous return of blood from the feet. Again the pressure effects of gravity are essentially proportional to a column of blood of a length equal to the distance from the level of the heart or the phlebostatic level to the vein under consideration. For example, if a vein in the foot of a normal man who is standing still is 120 cm. below the level of the right atrium, the pressure influence of gravity is equal to a column of 1200 mm. of blood. The pressure in the capillaries of his feet, therefore, must be at least of that magnitude, which is usually more than the pressure in the arteries of the man's arm. Thus energy sufficient to overcome this force must be supplied in order to re-establish and to maintain venous return to the heart. Since the arterial and venous systems are continuous, they may be considered to be U-tubes (Fig. 61). The force of gravity increases the pressure head on the arterial

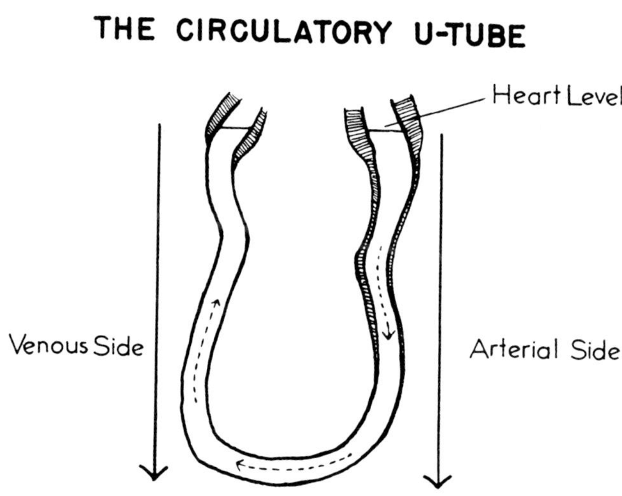

FIG. 61.—Arterial and venous sides of circulation form a U-tube, such as is indicated in this illustration for a man standing.

side by an amount equal to the retarding influence of gravitational force on the venous side. The net effect is essentially one of increasing the pressure in the vascular systems, distending the vessels, and increasing the volume of blood within these vessels.

Even though the energetic influences of the hydrostatic force of gravity tend to be equalized when the arterial and venous systems are considered, the net result is for the venous circulation to be impaired or to be at a disadvantage because of the mass of blood accumulated in the tissues below the level of the heart as well as the high pressure and distention of the veins.

Also in response to these high pressures the arterioles constrict, and pulsatile phenomena are impaired by this vasoconstriction and by stretching of the walls of the vessels, especially of the veins. Therefore, when the position of the body as a whole or any of its parts is changed, the gravitational influences will either impair or facilitate venous return, depending on whether or not the veins under consideration at the moment are below or above the level of the heart.

6) **Relative Volume of Blood in the Arterial and Venous Systems.**—The amount of blood entering the capillaries and veins from the arterial side of

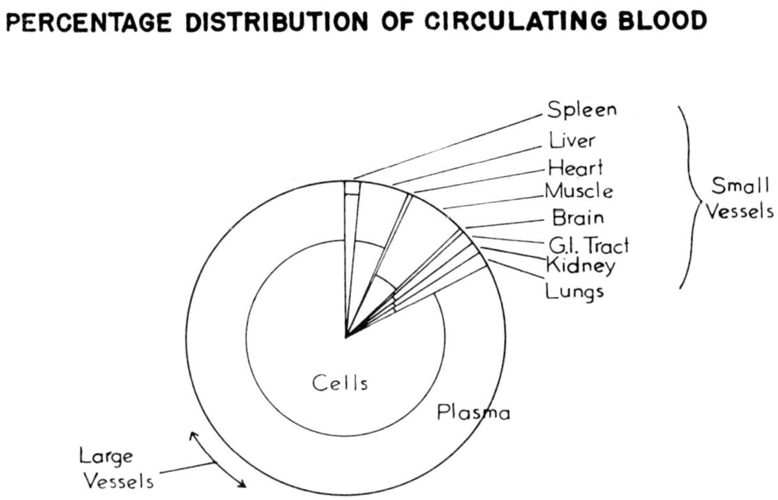

FIG. 62.—Diagrammatic representation of the apparent distribution of the blood in the circulating system of man. (Modified from the studies in dogs of Gibson and his associates, J. Clin. Investigation, *25*: 848, 1946.)

the circulation determines the pressure within them. The greater the volume of blood entering the venous system, the higher will be the venous pressure and the more effective will be venous return of blood. Obviously, there cannot be any disproportion for prolonged periods between cardiac output, or rate of volume flow in the arterial system, and rate of cardiac inflow, or rate of volume flow in the venous system, without disturbance in hemodynamics. With arteriolar constriction, everything else remaining constant, the rate of volume flow into the venous system is reduced and so also is the volume of blood within it reduced slightly. This slight decrease in venous blood volume and loss of *vis a tergo* results in lowering of venous pressure and, therefore, reduction in the rate of venous return. If this should persist, shock would ensue. Arteriolar dilatation, on the other hand, accelerates the rate of volume flow into the venous system, producing possibly a slight increase in venous pressure and greater increase in rate of venous return of blood to the heart.

If the volume of blood in the veins increases, there is usually an increased total blood volume, and since the veins serve as the main blood reservoir (Fig. 62), an increase in venous blood volume produces an increase in venous pressure (Fig. 63). Within limits the venous system may increase in

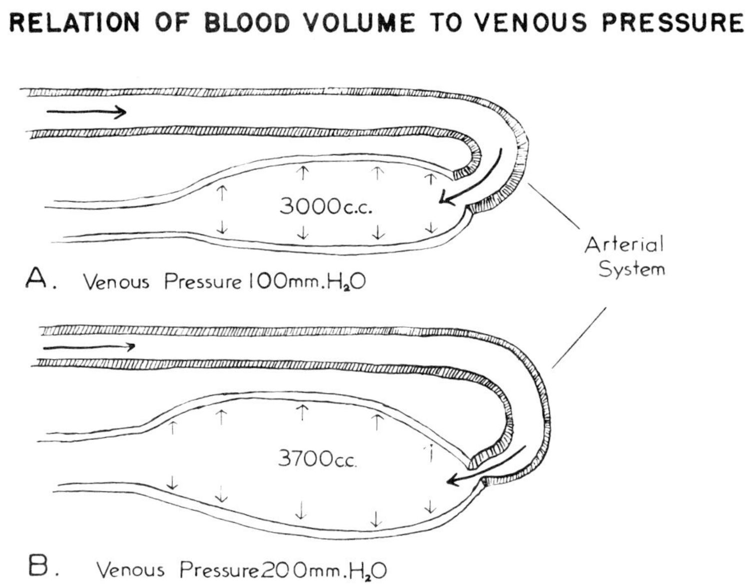

FIG. 63.—Influence of blood volume in venous system on venous pressure. *A* Essentially normal relationship. *B*, Venous blood volume increased; consequently the venous pressure is increased.

volume without venous pressure being elevated, since the veins distend easily (Fig. 64). However, after a certain amount of distention further increase in volume of blood within the veins produces a fairly rapid rise in venous pressure (Fig. 64), since the walls of the veins must be stretched to accommodate the additional volume of blood. The stretched walls offer a counterforce against the blood contained within the veins, and the intraluminal pressure is thus elevated.

RELATIONSHIP OF VENOUS PRESSURE TO VOLUME

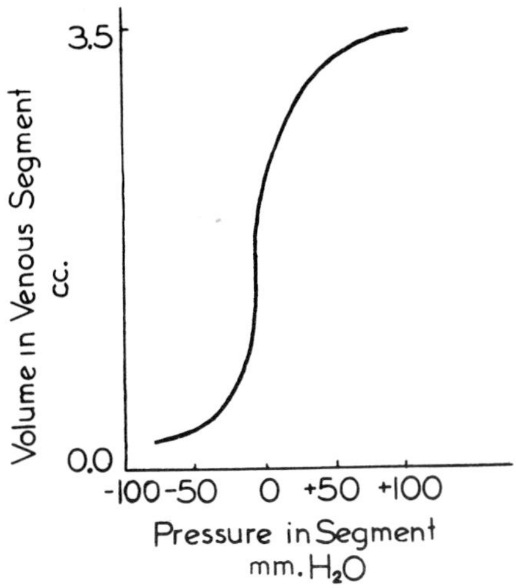

FIG. 64.—Relationship of the volume of blood in a vein to its venous pressure. The volume of a vein may be increased slightly without much change in venous pressure because of the ease of distensibility of the venous wall. However, as this distensibility is lost, a unit change in volume produces a great rise in venous pressure, until overstretching occurs. (Modified from Ryder *et al.*, J. Clin. Investigation, *23*, 355, 1944.)

7) **Venous Tone.**—The tone, tightness or state of constriction of the walls of the veins upon the blood contained therein, influences the venous pressure and pressure head, and, therefore, the rate of return flow of blood to the heart. Veins in a state of constriction tend to have higher pressure than when relaxed or "dilated," all other factors being equal (Fig. 65). Since the tone of veins, like the tone of arteries, is dependent upon sympathetic nervous and certain humoral influences, venous pressure becomes a partial index of sympathetic nervous or humoral activity.

VENOUS TONE AND VENOUS PRESSURE

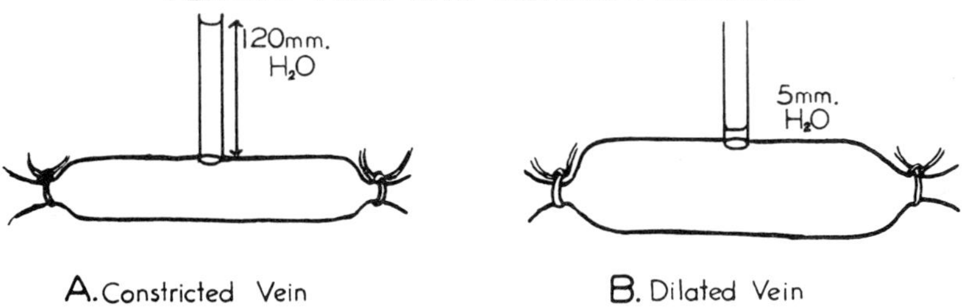

FIG. 65.—A constricted vein, *A*, has a higher venous pressure than a dilated or relaxed one, *B*.

Sudden decline in tone locally or generally is responsible for local or general venous stasis and impaired venous return of blood to the heart. Venous pressure changes locally or generally accordingly. Local loss in tone disturbs blood flow within a limited amount of tissue, but a general reduction impairs cardiac output and circulation throughout the body, so that circulatory collapse or shock follows.

FLOW OF BLOOD IN VEINS

The flow of blood in veins, because of lower pressure levels and less rapid linear rates of flow, tends to be different from that in arteries. Some of these differences are discussed briefly.

Streamline Flow.—Blood flowing into a collecting vein or blood flowing into a larger vein formed by the union of two or more veins tends to remain in separate streams for a considerable length of time before mixing (Fig. 66). Such respective streams have been traced by means of dyes. In

STREAMLINE FLOW

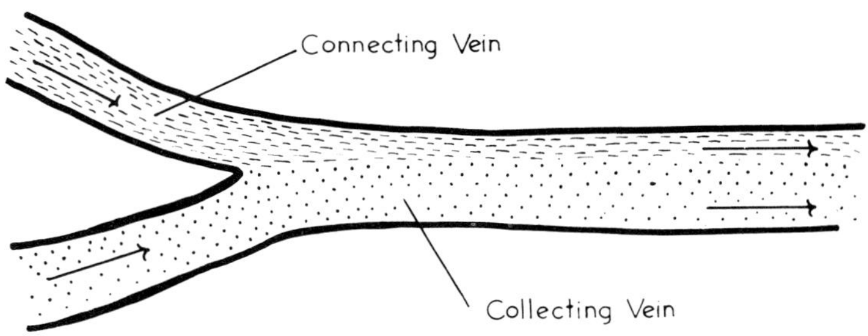

FIG. 66.—Streamline flow is evident by the fact that blood from a connecting vein does not mix with that of a collecting vein. The linear rate of flow is relatively slow in veins and, therefore, turbulence is less likely to exist.

arteries, where pressure gradients are relatively large, streamline flow is not as likely to occur, as turbulence and eddy currents at the points of junction of these vessels facilitate immediate mixing of the blood from the different vessels. This is also true for veins in which the rate of flow is rapid, such as in those of an elevated arm (Fig. 67). More important still, a single artery bifurcates into smaller ones, whereas veins collect into larger ones. Streamline flow would be more likely to occur where vessels collect into larger ones (Fig. 66) and where the rate of blood flow is slow enough so as not to produce turbulence. With streamline flow and turbulence tending to occur near the points of junction of veins, it is preferable, therefore, to lect for measurements of venous pressure sites of veins which are as far away as possible from points of junction. This may not *always* be feasible or even desirable, but these phenomena and their effects should be taken into consideration.

Backward Flow.—In a network of small veins in particular, as well as in larger ones, backward flow occurs as a result of changes in direction of pressure gradients. This phenomenon is important physiologically and

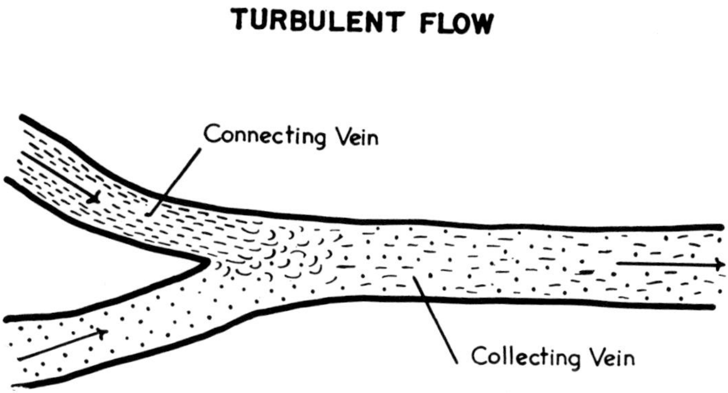

Fig. 67.—Absence of streamline flow in veins in which the linear rate of flow is relatively high and turbulence occurs at the junction of the vessels so that mixing results.

clinically. Frequently it occurs spontaneously or is present at times within some networks of veins. This has been observed by capillaroscopy (Fig. 68). Backward flow is likely to occur in certain disease states, for example, valvular incompetence or venous obstruction. In patients with incompetent valves associated with varicosities of the lower extremities there is

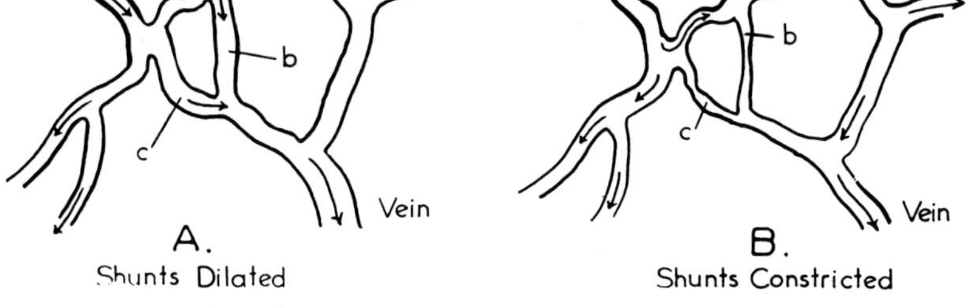

Fig. 68.—Reversal of flow in a given vessel. *A* shows blood flowing in vessel *a* from right to left, whereas *B* shows blood flowing in the opposite direction in vessel at a later time because of vasoconstriction of vessels *b* and *c*.

reversal of flow. Part (*A*) of Figure 69 shows a segment of deep and superficial veins of the leg joined by a communicating vein in which all valves are competent. Under such circumstances blood can flow only in one direction through the communicating vein—from the superficial veins to the deep. Part (*B*) of Figure 69 shows the influence of an incompetent valve in the

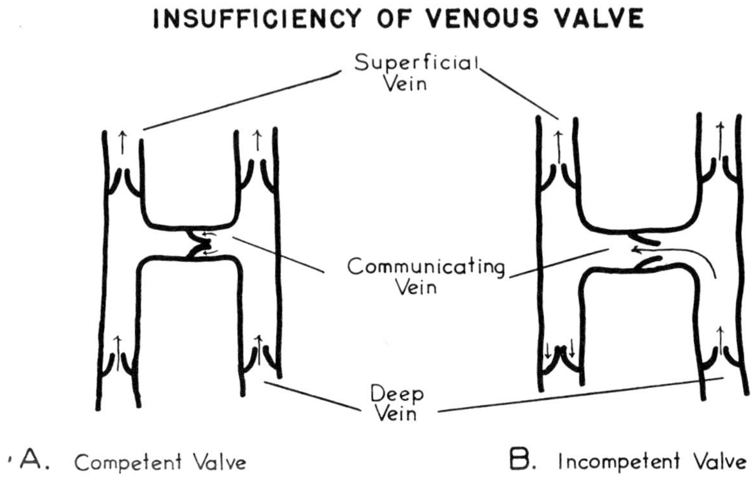

Fig. 69.—Segment of deep and superficial veins of leg with a communicating vein. *A*, Valves competent with unidirectional flow in all veins shown, including the communicating vein. *B*, Valves of communicating vein incompetent and flow is therefore possible in either direction, the direction of flow depending on the relative levels of pressure in the superficial and deep veins at that time.

communicating vein produced by abnormal dilatation of that vein. Blood may flow back and forth from the superficial to the deep vein. The significance of such a phenomenon is well known in the management of varicose veins.

Another example of backward flow is that encountered in veins obstructed by lesions. An excellent illustration of this is obstruction to the inferior vena cava (Fig. 70). Normally, with a fully patent inferior vena cava, blood flows from the inferior epigastric vein into the inferior vena cava (Fig. 70 *A*). When the latter is obstructed, the direction of flow is reversed, or the inferior epigastric vein becomes a collateral venous channel. This phenomenon is valuable in clinical diagnosis. Many other instances of backward flow in veins in disease states are well known and, therefore, need not be discussed.

ARTERIOVENOUS COMMUNICATIONS

Arteriovenous communications are of both physiologic and clinical interest. Certain aspects of these communications which are of general

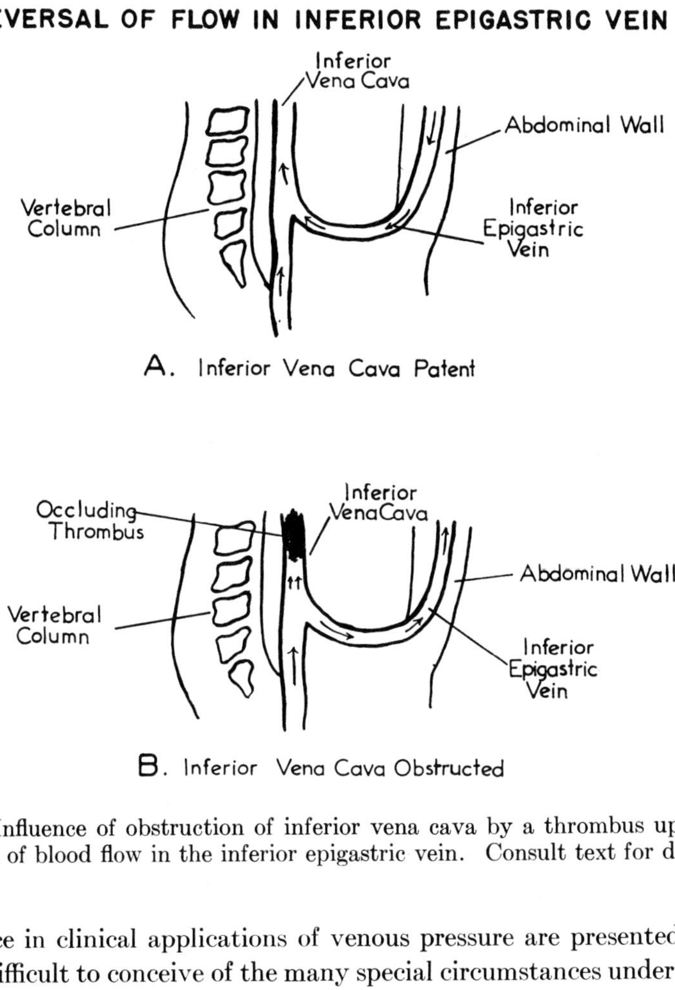

Fig. 70.—Influence of obstruction of inferior vena cava by a thrombus upon the direction of blood flow in the inferior epigastric vein. Consult text for details.

significance in clinical applications of venous pressure are presented here. It is not difficult to conceive of the many special circumstances under which such anastomoses are important clinically.

The influence of the special type of arteriovenous anastomosis or thoroughfare vessel in the villi of the intestine upon maintaining portal venous pressure and therefore flow has been indicated (Fig. 53, page 58). Another special type of anastomosis is that encountered in the peripheral circulation, namely, the thoroughfare vessels (Fig. 71) and glomus bodies. These anastomotic vessels are important in maintaining adequate circulation to the tissues in the periphery. The many complex aspects of their behavior will not be discussed. It is evident, however, that when these anastomotic vessels are wide open, the *vis a tergo* is transmitted directly into the small veins, thereby increasing the venous blood flow and venous pressure (Figure 71).

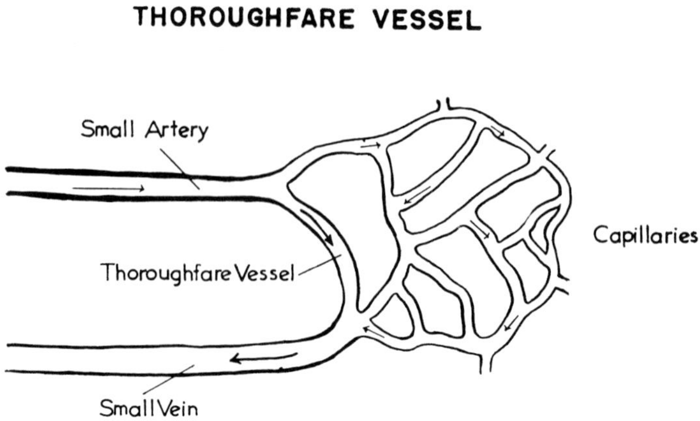

FIG. 71.—Thoroughfare vessel in the mesentery.

Abnormal arteriovenous anastomoses are extremely important in the application of determinations of venous pressure to clinical medicine. An appropriate example is the arteriovenous fistula which follows injury to veins and arteries adjacent to each other. Such an anastomosis between a large artery and vein permits direct transmission of arterial pressure and, of course, arterial blood into an adjacent vein (Fig. 72). The communication results in a local disturbance in venous flow and hemodynamics. Venous pressure is elevated in the region of the fistula by the arterial pressure

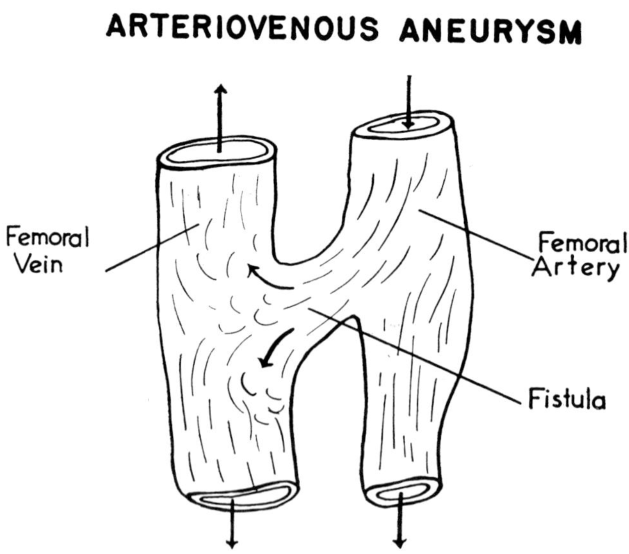

FIG. 72.—Arteriovenous aneurysm. Consult text for details.

transmitted therein. The high arterial pressure forces oxygenated blood into the venous system. Local pressure becomes sufficiently great to produce a backward flow in the adjacent group of veins and, likewise, to impair venous flow from tributaries emptying into the main collecting venous channels with the high pressure. Venous pressure is, therefore, elevated and the veins are distended. The veins appear less blue and more red. Turbulence of flow in the immediate vicinity of the fistulae produces a continuous machine-like murmur with exacerbations during systole. The venous pressure is pulsatile and varies considerably in closely adjacent areas because of the turbulence of flow and the relative influence of kinetic and

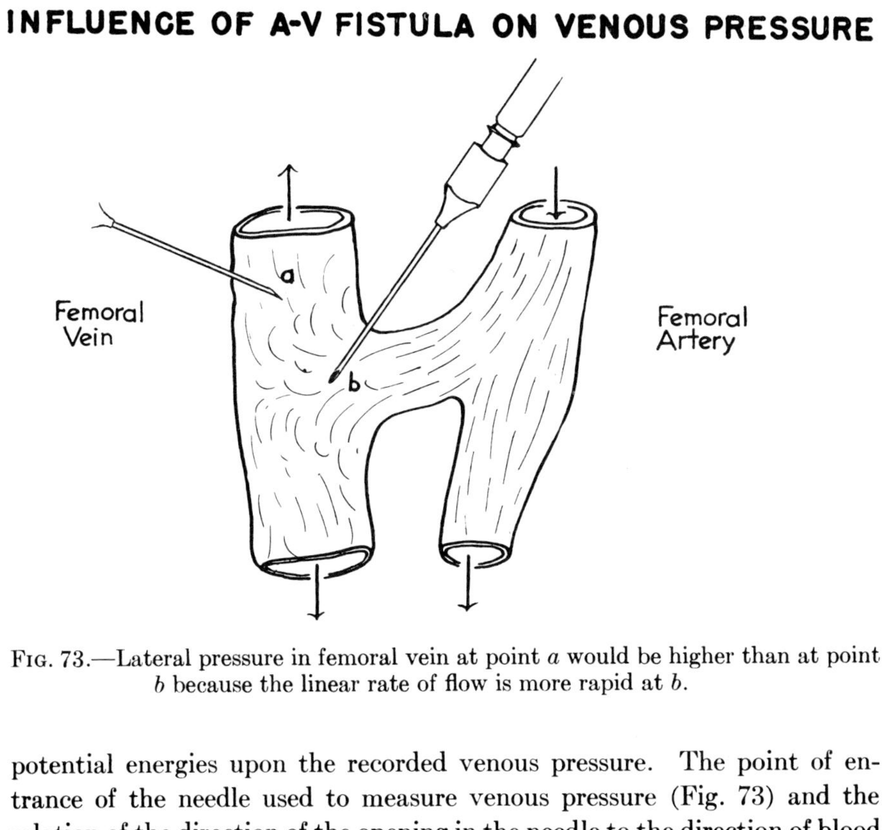

FIG. 73.—Lateral pressure in femoral vein at point *a* would be higher than at point *b* because the linear rate of flow is more rapid at *b*.

potential energies upon the recorded venous pressure. The point of entrance of the needle used to measure venous pressure (Fig. 73) and the relation of the direction of the opening in the needle to the direction of blood flow (Fig. 74) influence the results. These factors must be properly considered when venous pressure is being measured in the region of an arteriovenous aneurysm. They also explain the wide variations in values obtained in such a region, including cirsoid aneurysms or congenital arteriovenous anastomoses.

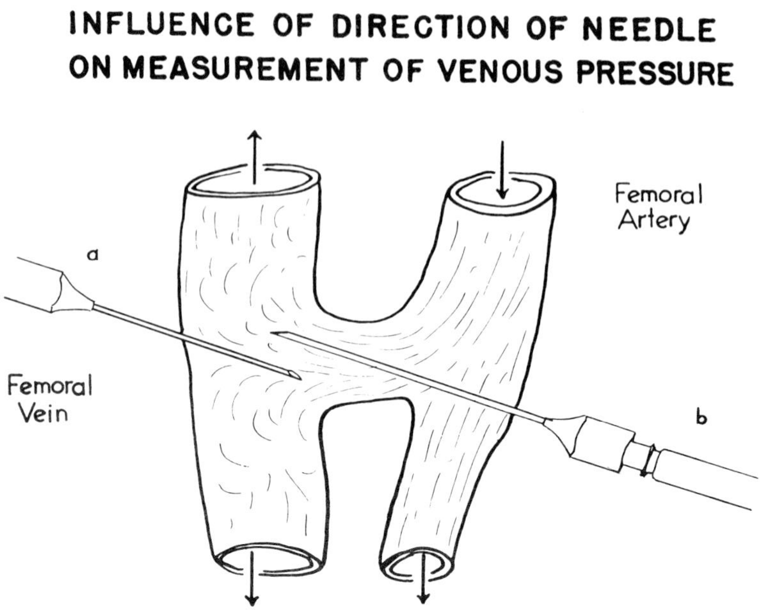

FIG. 74.—Influence of direction of needle opening and blood flow in region upon recorded venous pressure. A higher pressure would be recorded by needle *a* than *b*, since the effect of the kinetic energy of flow would be added to the force of the lateral pressure, whereas in needle *b* the effect of the kinetic energy would be subtracted from the lateral pressure.

PULSATIONS IN VENOUS PRESSURE

Pulsations in venous pressure vary in characteristics and are due largely to the following major factors:

1) ventricular systole
2) auricular and ventricular filling and emptying
3) respiration
4) noncardiac muscular contractions
5) contractions of the venous wall.

1) **Pulsations in Venous Pressure Due to Ventricular Systole.**—With each contraction of the ventricles a pulsatile variation in pressure may be transmitted directly into the small peripheral veins from the arterial side of the circulation (Fig. 75). This is particularly likely to occur if there is extreme peripheral dilatation, such as is encountered upon prolonged exposure to a hot and humid atmosphere. Variations in venous pressure which are synchronized with systolic and diastolic arterial pressures in the peripheral vessels can be recorded.

Pulsatile variations in venous pressure occur in veins which course adjacent to pulsating arteries. The pulsating wall of the artery presses upon

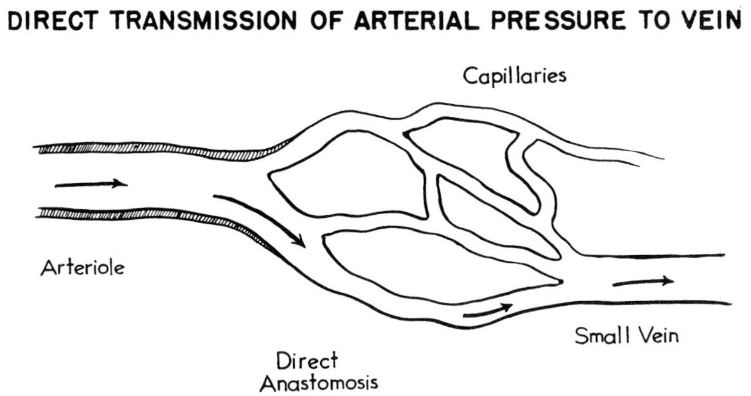

FIG. 75.—Dilatation of an arteriole and an arteriovenous communicating vessel permits the transmission of pulsatile variations in pressure into a small vein from the arterial side of the circulation.

the wall of the adjacent vein, compressing it and causing the pressure within to rise locally (Fig. 76). Because of competent venous valves this energy is transferred into unidirectionally active kinetic energy of flow, thus aiding in venous return (Fig. 76).

2) **Pulsation in Venous Pressure Due to Auricular and Ventricular Filling and Emptying.**—The influence of right atrial and ventricular filling and emptying upon the pressure within the external jugular vein is well exemplified by the well known jugulargram (Fig. 77). These variations in

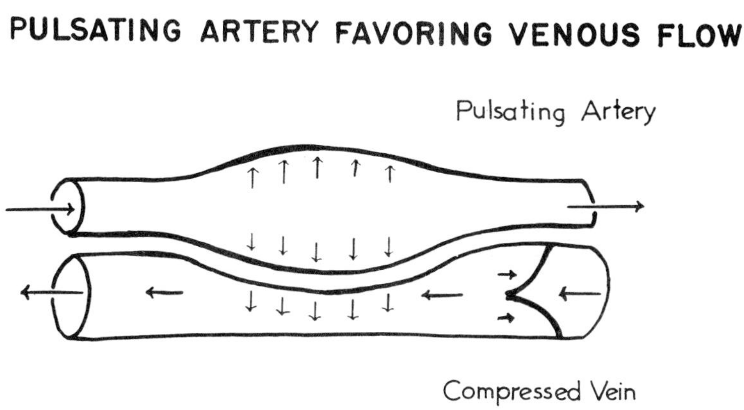

FIG. 76.—Artery transmitting pulsations in pressure to an adjacent vein by compressing it as the pulse wave travels by.

venous pressure are observed in vessels near the heart, especially the large tributaries of the superior and inferior vena cavae which empty into the vena cavae near the heart. Of diagnostic value is the fact that pathologic

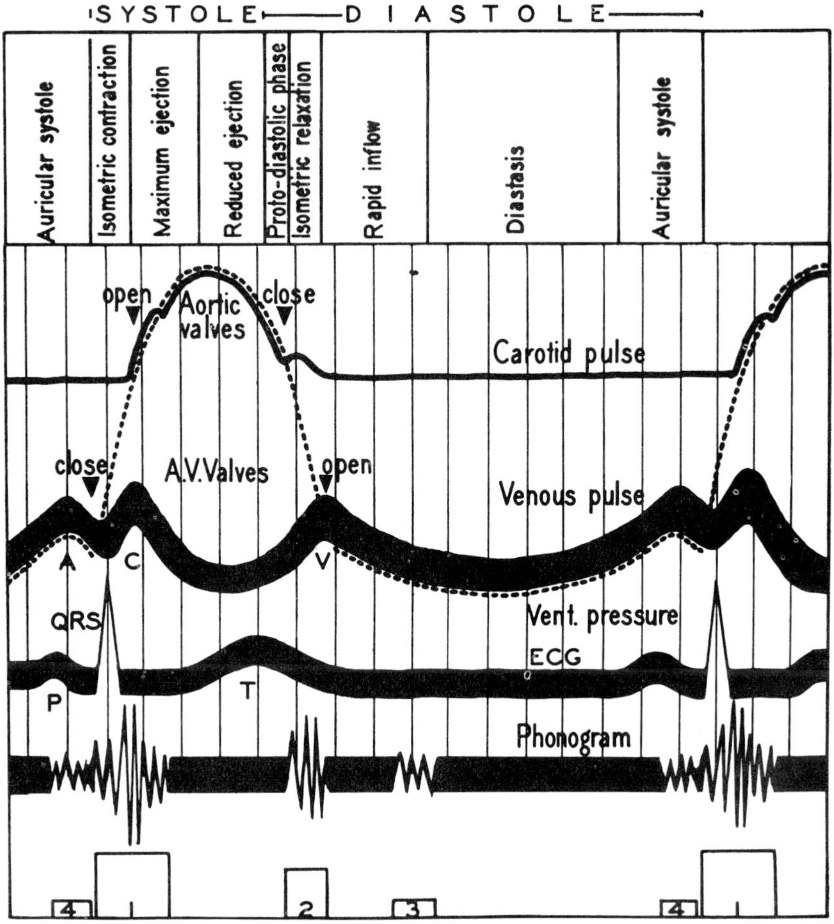

FIG. 77.—Diagram showing the relationship of the components of the phlebogram, heart sounds and other types of physical cardiovascular activities. (From Burch, G. E. and Reaser, P.: Primer of Cardiology, 1947, Lea and Febiger.)

states will alter these pulsations in pressure. They are usually determined by means of a recording of the jugular pulse but may be recorded by means of direct determinations of venous pressure.

3) **Pulsations in Venous Pressure Due to Respiration.**—The phases of respiration are associated with variations in intrathoracic pressure which influence venous pressure. The nearer the veins are to the thorax, the greater is the influence of respiration upon the pressure within the vein. As indicated previously, *inspiration* reduces the pressure of the veins within the thorax and of the veins draining into the superior vena cava, but the descending movement of the diaphragm with respiration increases intra-abdominal pressure and, therefore, the pressure within the veins of the abdomen and their tributaries. *Expiration* has the opposite effect; it increases the pressure within the veins in the thorax and their tributaries with the exception of the extrathoracic portions of the tributaries of the inferior vena cava but decreases the pressure within the intra-abdominal veins and their tributaries as the diaphragm elevates and reduces intra-abdominal pressure.

4) **Pulsation in Venous Pressure Due to Contraction of Noncardiac Muscle,** especially of skeletal muscle, produces variations in venous pressure. These changes are important in aiding venous blood flow to the heart and have been discussed in this Chapter.

5) **Pulsations in Venous Pressure Due to Contraction of the Venous Wall.**—Peristaltic waves within the arteries and veins have been described. These contractions increase venous pressure locally (Fig. 78) and, with the aid of competent valves, assist in venous flow of blood to the heart. These variations in venous pressure can be determined by direct methods of measurement.

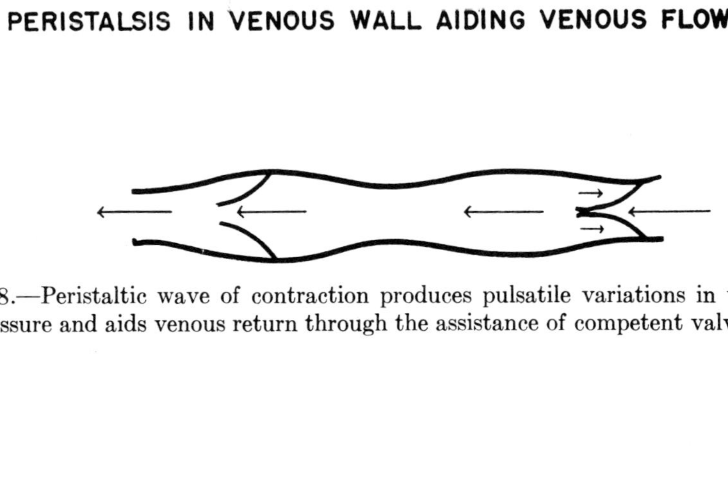

FIG. 78.—Peristaltic wave of contraction produces pulsatile variations in venous pressure and aids venous return through the assistance of competent valves.

CHAPTER 3

MEASUREMENT OF VENOUS PRESSURE

SINCE it is not the purpose of this presentation to discuss the various methods of recording venous pressure, only the general principles of the methods and a brief account of several of the most useful ones will be discussed. The methods employed for either clinical or experimental use must suit the needs of the study, but since most of them fail to fulfill all of the more important requirements, they have limited applications. Because the method involving the use of the phlebomanometer tends to achieve these requirements, it will be discussed in greatest detail. This apparatus offers certain definite advantages, especially its applicability to almost any visible vein in any part of the body. It should be possible to measure the pressure in a vein in any edematous area as well as in a median basilic vein. The procedure must be relatively simple to be practical clinically .The clinician should, of course, also be able to interpret the observations for the individual circumstances of measurement.

LEVEL OF REFERENCE

Before methods for measuring venous pressure or the normal and abnormal values are presented, "heart level" or the level of reference on which all measurements are based will be discussed. A dependable zero level of reference would be ideal—a level of reference comparable to "sea level" or "zero level" used in meteorologic or physics laboratories (Figs. 79 and 80).

SEA LEVEL

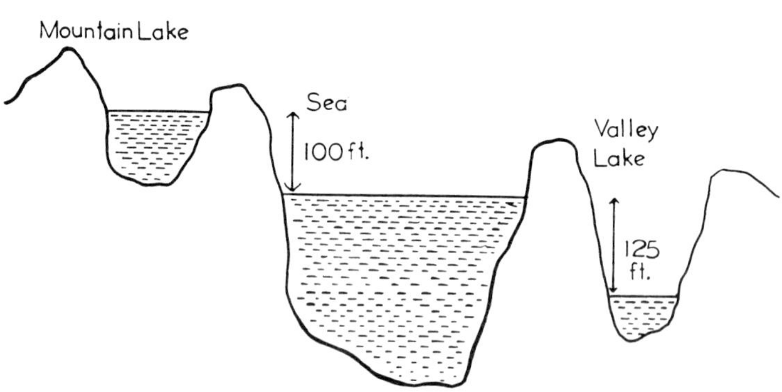

FIG. 79.—Level of sea is a reference level of measurements of altitude. Consult the text for details.

The geologist or meteorologist speaks of feet above or below sea level. For example, in Figure 79 the surface of the lake in the mountain is 100 feet above the level of the sea, a measurement of altitude. Since it is above the level of reference, it is said to have a *positive height* of 100 feet. The lake in the valley shown in Figure 79 has its surface 125 feet below the level of the sea and is therefore said to have a *negative height* of 125 feet. It is obvious that these values are relative. For example, the surface of the mountain lake would have a positive height of 225 feet and the sea level would have a positive height of 125 feet with respect to the surface of the lake in the valley. In physics laboratories or aviation a similar type of reference for pressure is employed; reference is made to the open atmosphere for barometric pressure, such as the sea and lake just described.

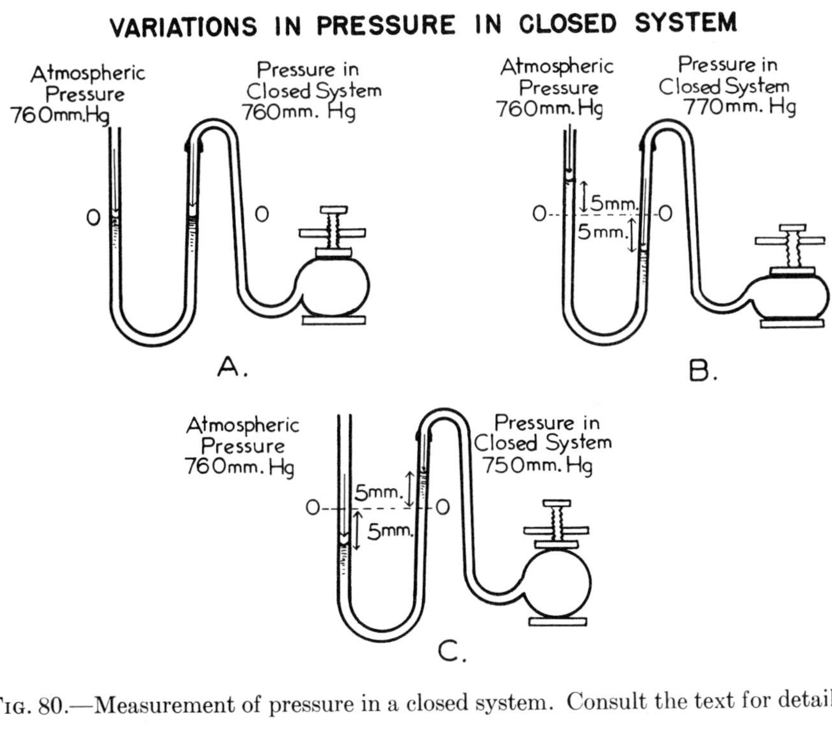

FIG. 80.—Measurement of pressure in a closed system. Consult the text for details.

When a closed system, such as the vascular system, including the veins, is under study, the reference level of pressure is also that of the atmosphere (Fig. 80). For example, in Figure 80 *A* the pressure within the system of the rubber pressure bulb, which is closed, is equal to the atmospheric pressure or 760 mm. of mercury. Thus the pressure acting on the surface of the left column of mercury is equal to that on the right column in the U-tube manometer. Therefore, the levels of the surfaces or heights of the two columns are equal. The pressure in the closed system is said to be *zero* or to have a zero difference from atmospheric pressure. In Figure 80 *B* the *screw clamp* has squeezed the rubber pressure bulb of the closed system, compressed the air within, and raised the pressure to a level greater than that of the atmosphere. This has lowered the column of mercury 5 mm. on the right side of the U-tube manometer and has elevated it 5 mm. on the left. The heights of the two columns of mercury differ by 10 mm., indicating that the absolute pressure within the closed system is 770 mm. of mercury or, relative to the atmosphere, it is 10 mm. of mercury above atmospheric pressure. There is a *positive* pressure of 10 mm. of mercury within the system. Figure 80 *C* shows the rubber pressure bulb released somewhat so that the air within the closed system is decompressed. Thus the pressure within the closed system is less than that in the atmosphere. The atmospheric pressure is now greater than that in the bulb and the column of mercury is displaced toward the lower pressure, that of the closed system.

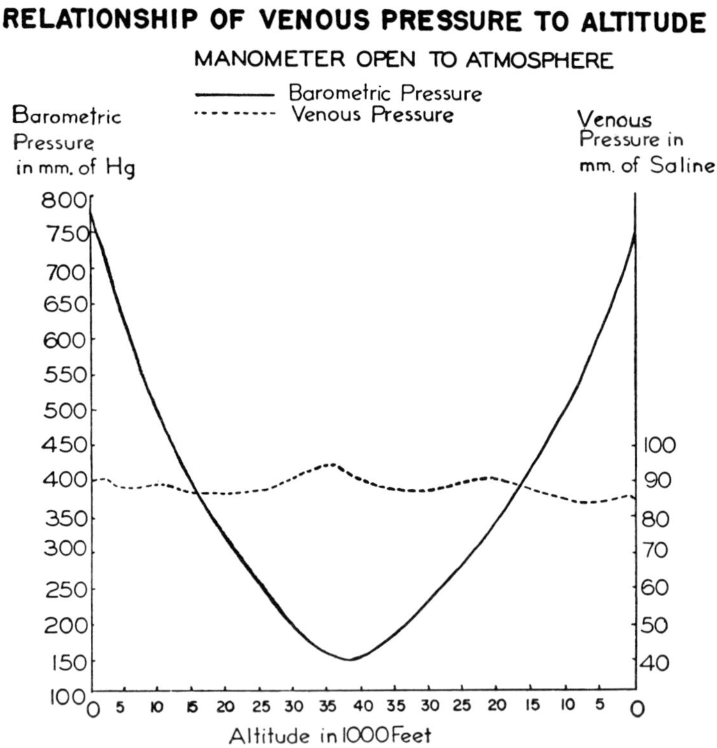

FIG. 81.—The venous pressure does not change, that is, it is essentially the same value above atmospheric pressure even with considerable changes in the latter. Since the pressures were measured with the manometers opened to the atmosphere, the venous pressure was compared with that in the atmosphere. (Courtesy of Sutherland *et al.*, J. Aviation Med., *14*, 280, 1943.)

Since the heights of the surfaces of mercury differ by 10 mm., the atmospheric pressure is 10 mm. of mercury above that in the closed system, or the pressure in the closed system in *minus* 10 mm. of mercury, relative to the atmosphere, or there is a negative pressure of 10 mm. of mercury in the closed system.

Since comparisons are made with respect to the atmospheric pressure and absolute pressure is not considered, it is not necessary to know the atmospheric pressure *per se* when venous pressure is being measured. For example, if the closed system illustrated in Figure 80 were the venous system, its pressure would be considered to be 0, + 10, and − 10 mm. of mercury respectively and *not* 760, 770 and 750 mm. of mercury. Therefore, since atmospheric pressure changes insignificantly during a brief period required for the measurement of venous pressure, the pressures recorded are those at, above or below that of the atmosphere.

The relationship of the pressure in the venous system to the atmospheric pressure is well illustrated by the changes in venous pressure with respect to

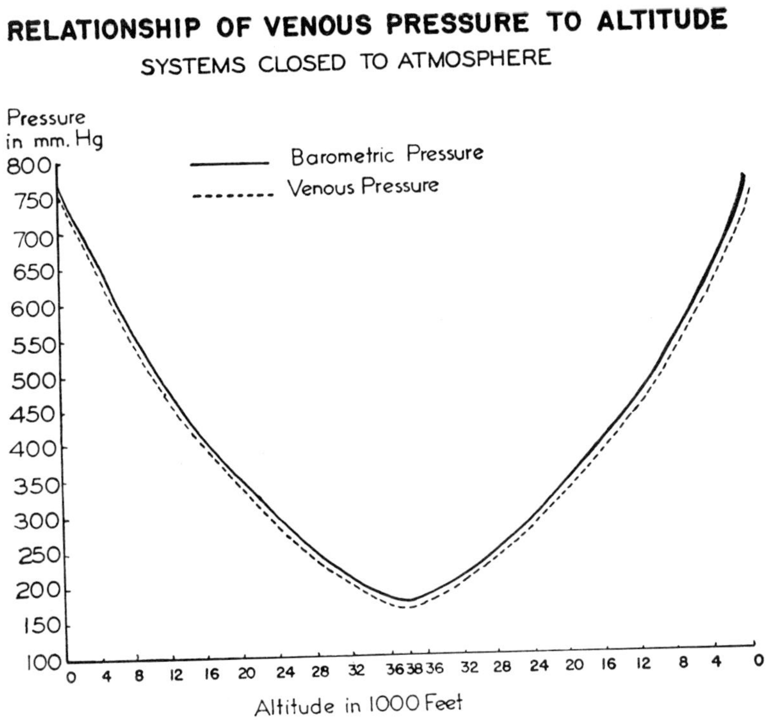

FIG. 82.—The absolute pressure in the venous system declines parallel to the decline in atmospheric pressure. This change in pressures or "absolute" pressures was measured with the manometers closed from the atmosphere. (Courtesy of Sutherland *et al.*, J. Aviation Med., *14*, 280, 1943.)

the change in atmospheric pressure occurring with increasing altitude. As a man ascends in an airplane, his venous pressure remains essentially at a constant level above that in the atmosphere (Fig. 81). However, as he ascends in the airplane, the *absolute* pressure in the veins declines parallel to that in the air (Fig. 82). Thus we see that with a manometer open to the atmosphere it is possible to compare automatically the pressure in a vein or any closed system with that in the atmosphere.

Influence of Gravity.—Since the venous system is closed, the pressure within the veins, like that within the remainder of the vascular system, is compared to that of the atmosphere. Therefore, when the pressure in a particular vein is determined, the reading obtained represents the pressure within that vein at that particular moment and for that particular position of the vein. However, the *force of gravity* offers another problem in the closed venous system. For example, the pressure within the veins of the hand is highest when the hand is hanging down at the subject's side and decreases as the hand is elevated (Fig. 83). If the hand is raised to the

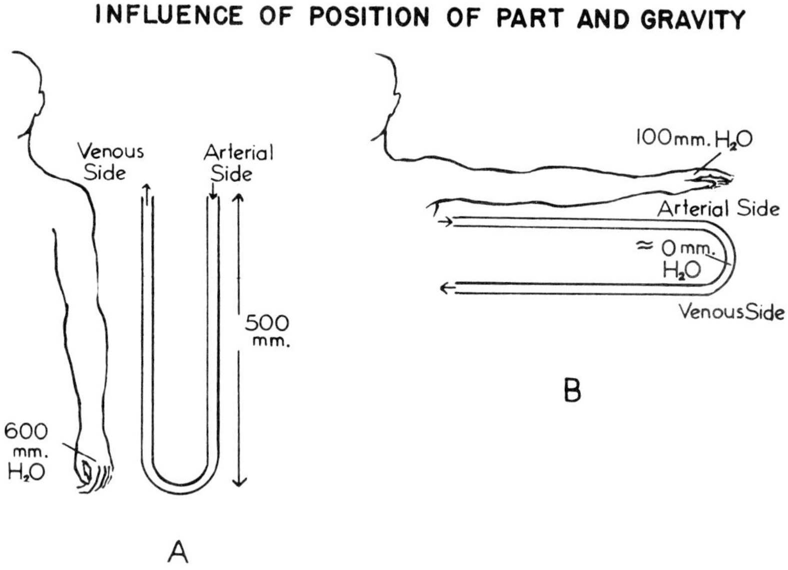

FIG. 83.—Influence of force of gravity upon pressure in veins of dorsum of hand. Consult the text for details.

level of the shoulder and the pressure within the veins of the dorsum of the hand is 100 mm. of water, this value indicates a pressure of 100 mm. of water above atmospheric pressure (Fig. 83 *B*).

The arterial and venous sides of the circulation may be considered as sides of a U-tube water manometer (Fig. 83), the specific gravity of the blood being assumed to be one for purposes of simplification. When the arm hangs down alongside the body, the pressure within the veins of the hand increases, because of the effect of gravity, by an amount equal to the length of the column of blood in the venous or arterial limb of the U-tube (Fig. 83). This is equal to the "weight" of the column of blood. Since the column is 500 mm. in length, the addition of the previous intrinsic pressure of 100 mm. of water yields a pressure of 600 mm. of water, the specific gravity of the blood being assumed to be one. Thus it is evident that the position of the vein under study or the influence of gravity upon the various columns of blood within the closed venous system will influence the level of pressure within a particular vein.

"Heart Level."—In order to overcome errors due to the influence of gravity, various investigators interested in the problem of venous pressure have attempted to find a point in the venous system at which the pressure is equal to that of the *atmosphere* or is *zero*. Many of them have considered this to be in the right atrium, although opinions have varied. Some observers consider it to be in the abdominal portion of the inferior vena cava, whereas others place it in the innominate vein near its junction with the external jugular vein. Sir Thomas Lewis designated the level of the suprasternal notch as the level of reference with the subject erect, but most observers have used the point of junction between the lateral border of the sternum and the fourth intercostal space. The latter point has been chosen because it is about the level at which the superior and inferior vena cavae enter the right atrium. When the subject is in the supine position, the point of reference employed has varied from within the most anterior to within the most posterior plane surface of the chest.

Phlebostatic Axis and Phlebostatic Level.—Since none of the points of reference is always at "zero" pressure or equal to atmospheric pressure, it is more important to employ a satisfactory standard level of reference which observers can learn to employ and with which they may become adequately acquainted to permit comparisons of values. For anatomic and physiologic reasons the concept of the (1) *phelbostatic axis* and (2) *phlebostatic level* was introduced. These terms, unlike the more specific "heart level" and "zero level," are not so definite, although objections have been voiced concerning the complexity of terminology. With continued use of the same level of reference observers become experienced in handling their data and in evaluating their significance so that satisfactory clinical and physiologic applications are possible.

1) *Phlebostatic axis* is defined as the *line of junction* between a transverse

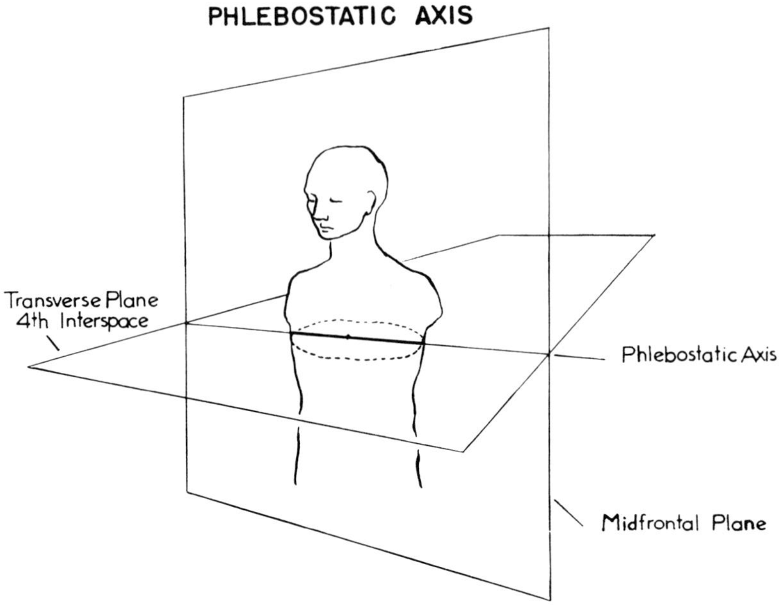

FIG. 84.—Phlebostatic axis.

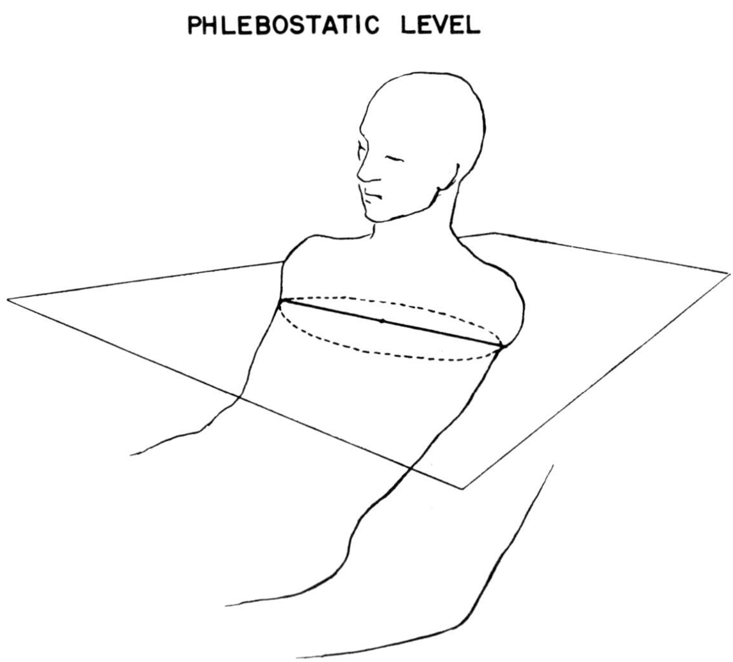

FIG. 85.—Phlebostatic level.

plane of the body passing through the points of junction of the lateral margins of the sternum and the fourth intercostal space and a frontal plane of the body passing through the midpoint of a line extending from the outermost point of the anterior surface of the sternum and the outermost point of the posterior surface of the chest (Fig. 84).

2) *Phlebostatic level* is defined as any plane which passes through the phlebostatic axis and is also parallel with the horizon (Fig. 85). No satisfactory level of reference has been described for use in a subject resting on one of his sides. The phlebostatic level is suggested as the level of reference and corresponds to the "heart level." Unfortunately, all venous pressures quoted from other observers in these discussions could not be corrected to this level of reference.

The phlebostatic level is infinite in extent, so that any vein in the body, regardless of its distance from the heart, can be referred to it. Furthermore, the phlebostatic level rotates about the phleobstatic axis as the subject changes from the supine to the erect position (Fig. 86). There is a need

BODY POSITION AND PHLEBOSTATIC LEVEL

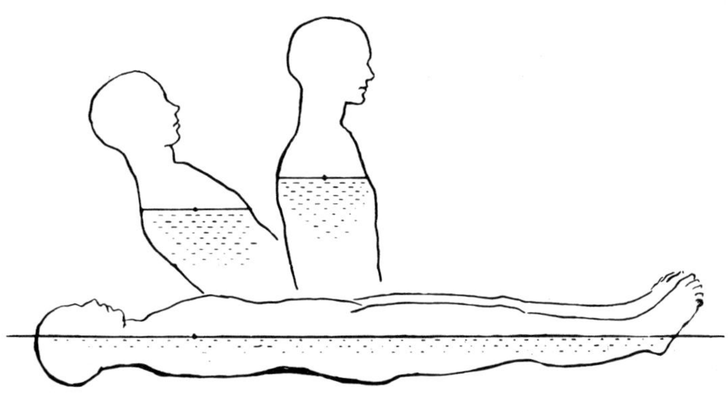

FIG. 86.—Rotation of phlebostatic level about the phlebostatic axis as a person sits erect or reclines.

for more studies to evaluate better the applicability of the phlebostatic level for various sitting positions.

It is well to note again that the phlebostatic level, like any other level of reference, is more or less arbitrary. Though it is based primarily upon an attempt to obtain a zero pressure level, it is actually determined by external anatomic or topographic landmarks and does not necessarily represent a level in the venous system where the pressure is equal to atmospheric pressure or is a true "zero" pressure level. Nevertheless, it is suitable for use in measurement of venous pressure and approaches zero pressure and is stable and reproducible.

The application of the phlebostatic level to variations in the position of the body from the supine to the sitting is illustrated by Figure 87. It is

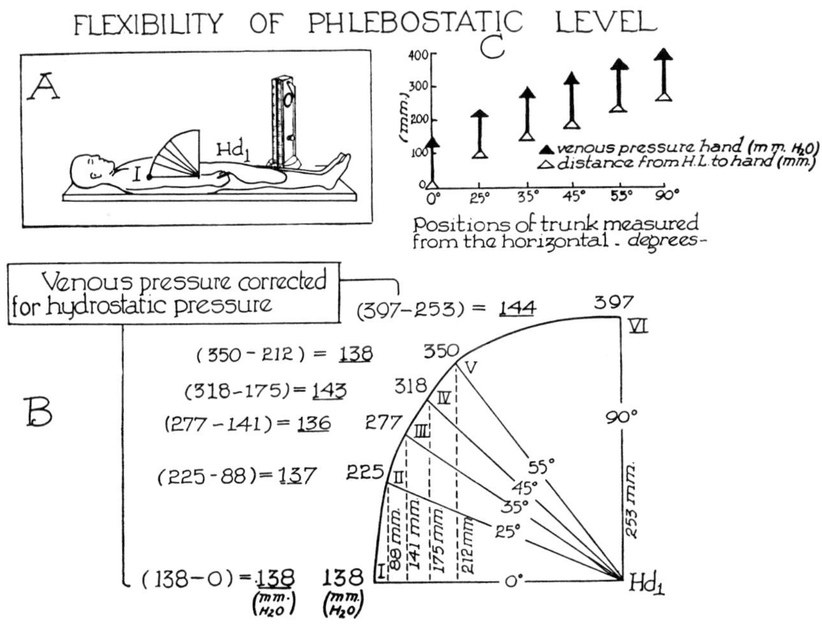

FIG. 87.—The phlebostatic level as the heart level in the supine, various intermediate sitting, and upright sitting positions. *A*, Subject in supine position and hand Hd_1 in horizontal plane passing through phlebostatic axis (black spot). Venous pressures corrected for hydrostatic pressure resulting from the elevation of the phlebostatic axis to Positions II, III, IV, V, and VI, leaving the hand in which venous pressure determination is being made in position Hd_1. *C*, Proportional increase in venous pressure and hydrostatic pressure with each change of trunk position. (From Winsor and Burch, Am. Heart J., *31*, 387, 1946).

evident from this figure that as body position changes and phlebostatic level is assumed to rotate about the phlebostatic axis in order to remain parallel to the horizon, the reference level remains dependable and suitable for application to the bedridden patient. Although this reference level may have certain disadvantages, it appears to be the most satisfactory for general purposes.

METHODS OF MEASURING VENOUS PRESSURE

Units of Venous Pressure

Because of the low pressures within the veins, measurements are expressed in millimeters of water. This should not be confused with the units used for arterial blood pressure, which is considerably higher and is expressed in millimeters of mercury. Since the specific gravity of mercury is approximately 13.5 times that of water, a pressure of 1 mm. of mercury is equal to a pressure of 13.5 mm. of water.

Since it is not possible to present all of the methods which have been introduced for the purposes of measuring venous pressure, only those which are most useful will be discussed.

Indirect Methods

a) **Method of Lewis.**—Sir Thomas Lewis pointed out that in the normal subject erect, the veins of the neck are collapsed. In persons with congestive heart failure and an elevation in venous pressure the external jugular vein is distended by the increased pressure within the veins (Fig. 88). Lewis also employed the vertical distance in millimeters from the

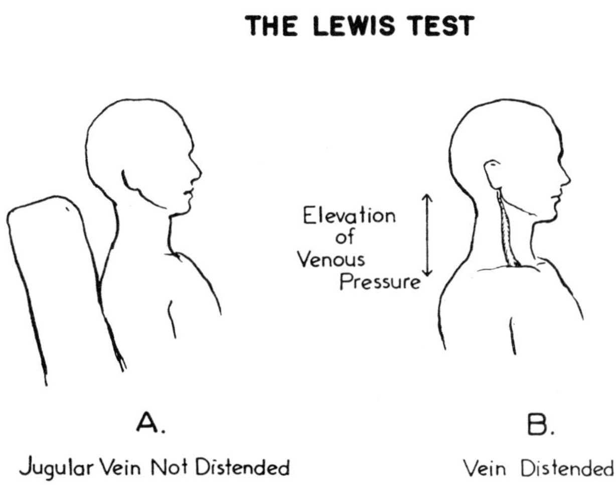

Fig. 88.—Measurement of venous pressure by method of Lewis. Consult the text for details.

suprasternal notch to the top of the column of blood visible in the external jugular vein as a measurement of the degree of elevation in venous pressure above normal in millimeters of blood or, for practical purposes, water. At least this observation should be employed routinely by all clinicians during careful physical examination of any patient. Unfortunately, the method is relatively inaccurate and measures only the pressure in the external jugular vein and is therefore inadequate though still useful at the bedside. In many instances the pressure in other veins should be measured, as that within the jugular vein is not necessarily an index of the pressure in the entire venous system.

b) **Method of Gaertner.**—Gaertner showed that the pressure in the veins of the dorsum of the hand of a subject may be estimated in the following manner. After the hand is allowed to hang down until its dorsal veins become distended with blood, the hand and elbow of the subject are rested upon the palms of the hands of the observer. They are gently raised by the observer (Fig. 89). The elevation is continued until the veins

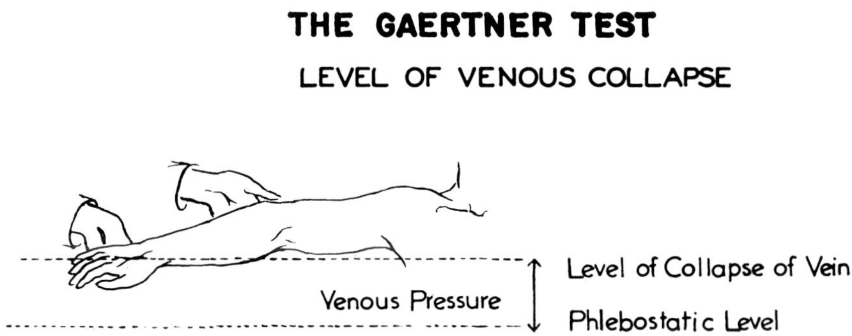

FIG. 89.—Measurement of venous pressure by method of Gaertner. Consult the text for details.

on the dorsal surface of the hand just collapse. The distance in millimeters from the phlebostatic level to the level at which a particular vein on the dorsum of the hand just collapses on elevation represents the venous pressure in millimeters of blood or, essentially, millimeters of water. Care must be taken to prevent constriction of the veins of the axilla by tight clothing, flexion of joints or muscular contraction.

Like the method of Lewis, the method of Gaertner is simple and requires no special apparatus. It is useful and is applied with success clinically when used intelligently. However, it is also subject to limitations, since it is indirect and may not be an index of the pressure within other portions of the venous system. Furthermore, it cannot be employed in a fat or edematous hand.

c) **Method of von Recklinghausen.**—The subject is made to lie in the supine position on a flat, firm examining table. One hand of the subject is placed upon his thigh and the other hand is placed alongside his body upon the examining table (Fig. 90). If the venous pressure is normal, the veins on the dorsum of the hand on the thigh will be collapsed while those on the dorsum of the hand on the table will be distended. If the veins on the dorsum of both hands are distended, then the venous pressure is abnormally elevated, and if they are collapsed on the dorsum of both hands, then the venous pressure is abnormally low. Care must be exercised to avoid constriction of veins by clothing, muscular contraction, or flexion at joints.

This method, like the two preceding, is indirect and may not indicate the pressure in other veins of the subject. Although it is not quantitative, it is easily applied at the bedside and requires no special apparatus.

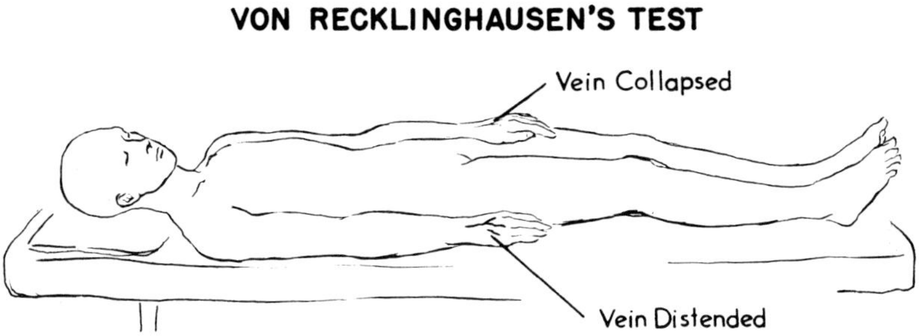

FIG. 90.—The method of von Recklinghausen.

DIRECT METHODS

Except for those just described, indirect methods for measurement of venous pressure are clinically impractical as well as inaccurate. Many procedures have been described for measuring venous pressure directly, most of which are based upon the method of Moritz and von Tabora (Fig. 91). The vein under study is punctured by a needle which is connected by means of rubber tubing to a glass column containing a physiologic solution of sodium chloride. This solution is allowed to run into the vein until the meniscus comes to a standstill. The distance in millimeters of the meniscus

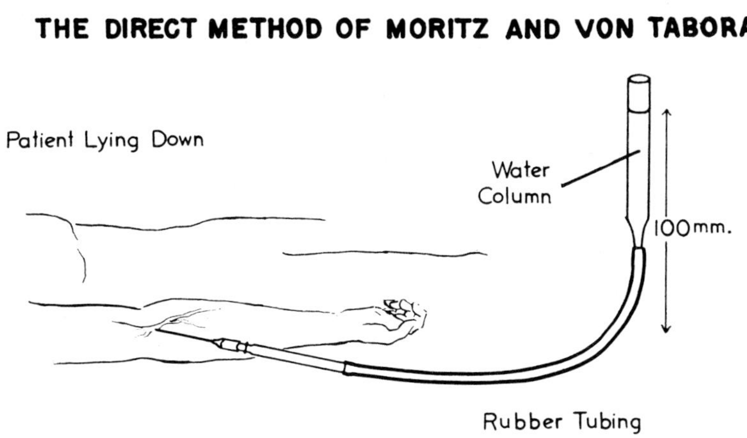

FIG. 91.—The method of Moritz and von Tabora, the fundamental direct method.

from the reference or "heart" level represents the pressure within the vein under study in millimeters of physiologic saline solution, or, for practical purposes, millimeters of water.

Obstruction of the needle by clotting, often overlooked, frequently offers difficulty. Flushing of the needle periodically will prevent clotting during prolonged periods of study. One of the disadvantages of this method is that it requires a large needle and therefore can be applied only to relatively large veins. Furthermore, the fluid injected into the subject may cause physiologic changes. It is also relatively painful. Other reasons for its impracticability include the fact that the entire apparatus must be sterilized and a fairly large amount of equipment must be balanced at the cardiac level.

The Phlebomanometer

The phlebomanometer is an instrument for the direct measurement of venous pressure. It is based upon well established principles of physics and physiology and has been employed in some form or another for the determination of pressure in blood vessels, tissues or body cavities. Because the method appears to offer advantages and because of the author's experience with the method, a detailed description of the apparatus and its use is included.

Essential Parts.—The apparatus, which is illustrated in Figures 92 and 93, consists essentially of three parts, a water manometer, a pressure bulb and a glass adapter or glass observation tube (Figs. 92 and 93). A three-way selector valve is provided, so that the pressure bulb and manometer, or observation tube and pressure bulb, or observation tube, manometer and pressure bulb may be connected. The glass observation tube (approximately 12 cm. long with a bore of 1.0 mm.), hypodermic needle and the 2 per cent aqueous solution of sodium citrate are the only portions of the apparatus which are sterilized, so that preparation and maintenance of the apparatus is relatively simple.

Use of the Phlebomanometer.—When placed in use the reservoir (Fig. 93) must contain clean water in an amount sufficient to reach the zero level. During transportation of the apparatus beads of water may accumulate in the tube of the manometer. These are removed by moving the selector valve to the position which connects only the manometer to the pressure bulb (Fig. 93). Thus it is possible to clear any beads of water out of the manometer column by turning the screw controlling the pressure bulb back and forth. *At this time it is important to make sure that the pressure*

ESSENTIAL PARTS OF THE PHLEBOMANOMETER

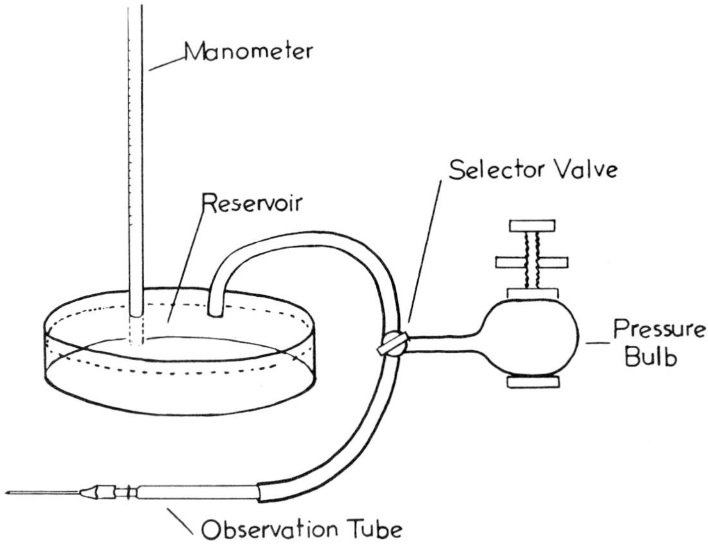

FIG. 92.—Diagram of the essential components of the phlebomanometer.*

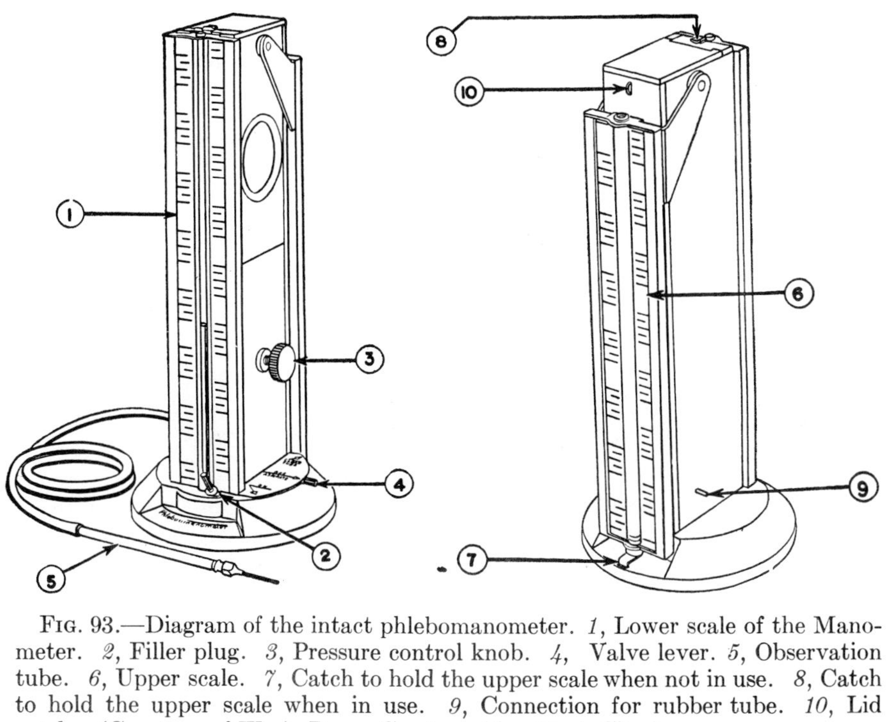

FIG. 93.—Diagram of the intact phlebomanometer. *1*, Lower scale of the Manometer. *2*, Filler plug. *3*, Pressure control knob. *4*, Valve lever. *5*, Observation tube. *6*, Upper scale. *7*, Catch to hold the upper scale when not in use. *8*, Catch to hold the upper scale when in use. *9*, Connection for rubber tube. *10*, Lid catch. (Courtesy of W. A. Baum Co. Inc., New York City.)

* This unit is manufactured by W. A. Baum Co. Inc. of New York.

bulb is partially compressed before the next phase of the procedure is undertaken.

The selector valve is then set to connect only the observation tube to the pressure bulb. This makes it possible to produce a negative pressure within the system in order to draw a column of the solution of 2 per cent sodium citrate into the observation tube. This could not be done without a valve when the straight single column type of manometer is used. A valve would not be necessary for a U-tube manometer. With the selector valve in this position, the tip of the needle connected to the observation tube is placed in an ampoule of sterile 2 per cent aqueous solution of sodium citrate and the knob (Fig. 93) controlling the pressure bulb is gradually unscrewed. A column of the solution of citrate is slowly drawn into the glass observation tube until the meniscus of the citrate solution reaches the region of the transverse lines on the observation tube (Fig. 94). It is *important* to re-

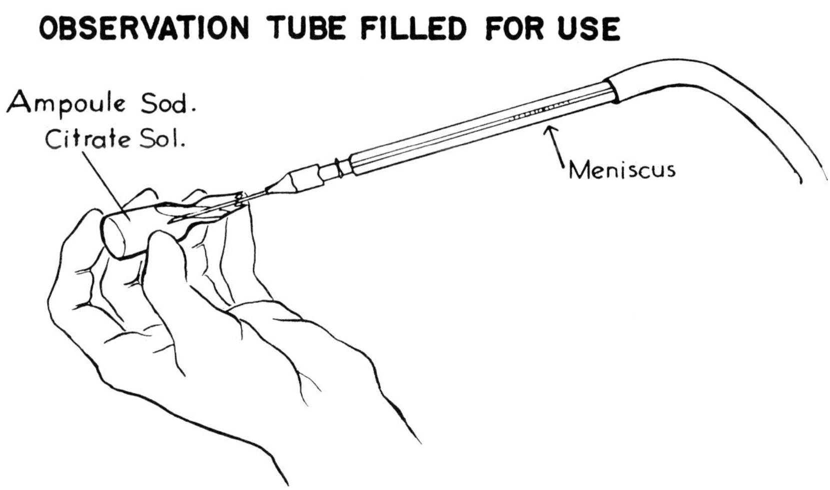

FIG. 94.—Observation tube with a column of solution of sodium citrate drawn into place with the meniscus at the level of the transverse lines on the tube.

member to screw the pressure bulb until the meniscus of the citrate solution is brought to a standstill before the tip of the hypodermic needle is removed from below the surface of the sodium citrate in the ampoule. If this precaution is not taken, air bubbles will be suddenly drawn into the observation tube and rubber tubing by the negative pressure created in the system by the pressure bulb, and the beads of citrate solution will have to be blown out of the system before the procedure can be begun again.

After the solution of sodium citrate has been properly drawn into the observation tube, the selector valve is moved to connect the manometer, pressure bulb and observation tube by means of the pneumatic system. The vein selected for study is brought to the phlebostatic level, if possible. If this is not possible, its position with respect to the phlebostatic level is noted in millimeters. When the vein is punctured with the hypodermic needle, the pressure within the vein will begin to force blood into the observation tube, which in turn will force the meniscus of the solution further up into the observation tube. Immediately after the vein is entered, the knob controlling the pressure bulb is screwed in to raise the pressure within the pneumatic system gradually until the meniscus of the solution of citrate is brought to a standstill. When this occurs, the pressure in the manometer is equal to the pressure in the vein; the pressure indicated on the manometer then represents the venous pressure.

As a check of the value obtained, it is advisable to lower or elevate the pressure within the pressure bulb to disturb the equilibrium, so that the meniscus moves again and the venous pressure may again be determined. These two values should agree within 2 or 3 millimeters of water.

After the needle is withdrawn, it is advisable to allow the citrate solution in the observation tube to flush the blood out of the needle in order to prevent a clot of blood from obstructing the needle during further use.

Correction for Capillarity in Observation Tube.—The capillarity of the observation tube is approximately 20 mm. of water. An automatic correction is made by holding the observation tube at a slight inclination with the index finger (Fig. 95) so that the meniscus of the citrate column in the

METHOD OF CORRECTING FOR CAPILLARITY IN OBSERVATION TUBE

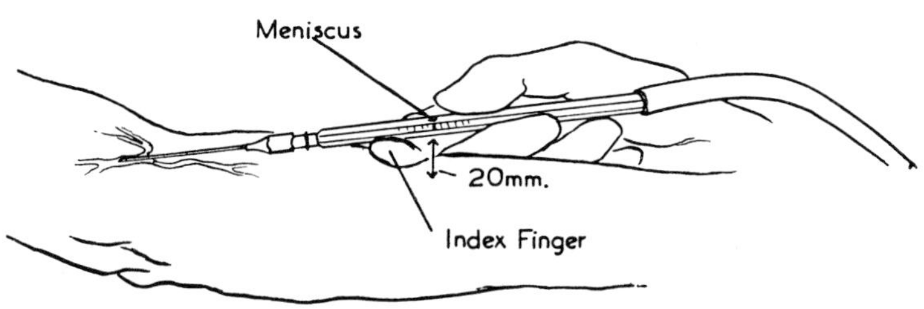

FIG. 95.—Method of automatically correcting for capillarity in observation tube With practice it is possible to insert the needle into the vein with the observation tube resting on the tip of the index finger so that the distance from the meniscus to the vein punctured is equal to the force of capillarity of the observation tube.

tube is about 20 mm. above the site of puncture of the vein. When it is not possible to puncture a vein in this manner, corrections must be made mathematically (Fig. 96).

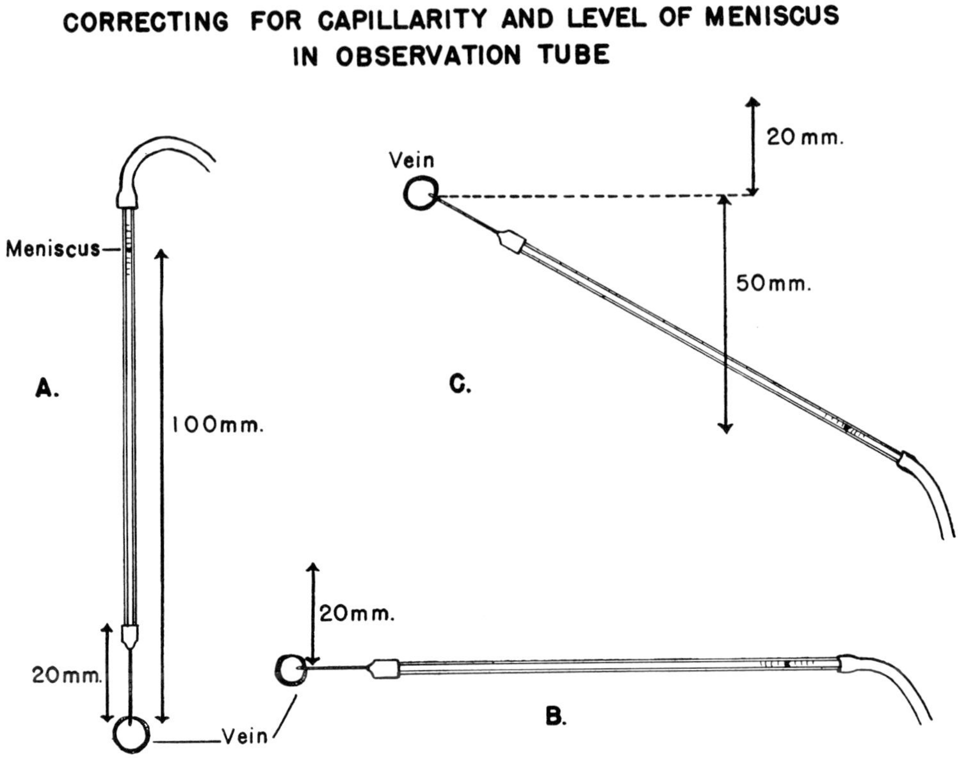

FIG. 96.—Method of correcting for capillarity when a vein is punctured in various directions so that the meniscus of the solution of sodium citrate is above, *A*, on the level with, *B*, or below, *C*, the vein under study.

Example 1.—When the meniscus of the citrate column in the observation tube is more than 20 mm. above the vein, the venous pressure in millimeters of water (Fig. 96 *A*) is expressed as follows:

Venous Pressure = Manometer value + (Distance of meniscus above vein in mm. − 20 mm.)

Therefore, in Figure 96 *A*,

Venous Pressure = Manometer value + (100 − 20) or
= Manometer value + 80.

Example 2.—When the pressure is measured so that the vein is punctured in such a manner that the meniscus of the citrate is on a level horizontal with the vein (Fig. 96 *B*), the venous pressure in millimeters of water is expressed as follows:

Venous Pressure = Manometer value − 20 mm.

Example 3.—When the pressure is measured so that the vein is punctured in such a manner that the meniscus of the citrate column is below the level of the vein (Fig. 96 *C*), the venous pressure in millimeters of water is expressed as:

Venous Pressure = Manometer value − (Distance of meniscus below vein in mm. + 20 mm.)

or in the example shown (Fig. 96 *C*) the venous pressure in millimeters of water would be:

Venous Pressure = Manometer value − (50 + 20 mm.)
= Manometer value − 70 mm.

The Observation Tube.—(*a*) *Amount of Fluid Involved.*—Because of the narrow bore (about 1.0 mm. in diameter) of the observation tube, only a small quantity of fluid, about 0.1 cc., is involved in a measurement of venous pressure. Therefore, an insignificant amount of blood is removed from the subject and little fluid is injected into him during a measurement. Physiologic alterations, as a result of disturbance in fluid volume, are therefore minimal—a decided advantage.

b) *Transverse Lines.*—The transverse lines provided on the observation tube aid in detecting slight movement of the meniscus. In determination of venous pressure it is necessary to make certain that the meniscus of the citrate is at a standstill or that the venous pressure is balanced. The finer the needle employed, the more caution must be taken to obtain complete immobility of the meniscus. The transverse lines are of assistance in achieving this (Fig. 97).

TRANSVERSE LINES OF OBSERVATION TUBE

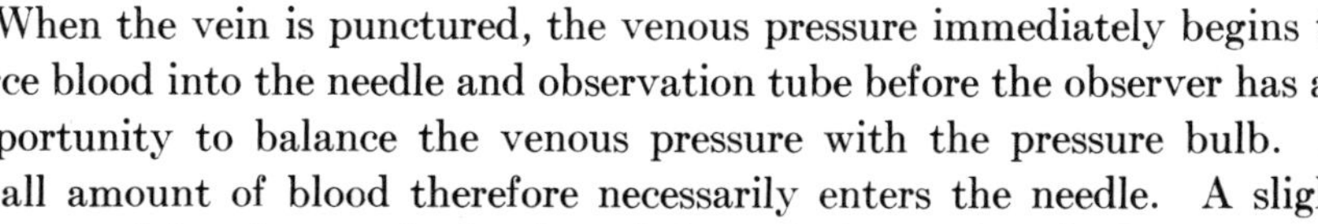

FIG. 97.—Transverse lines aid in detecting slight movement of meniscus.

When the vein is punctured, the venous pressure immediately begins to force blood into the needle and observation tube before the observer has an opportunity to balance the venous pressure with the pressure bulb. A small amount of blood therefore necessarily enters the needle. A slight amount of the citrate solution forced through the needle will flush out this blood (Fig. 98). The transverse lines aid in determining when the blood has been reinjected into the subject; when the meniscus returns to its previous position with respect to these transverse lines, most of the blood has been returned to the vein. Furthermore, during prolonged observations citrate solution should be flushed through the needle periodically to avoid clotting within it.

c) *Size of Observation Tube.*—The observation tube and needle are approximately the size of those of a tuberculin syringe, with which all doctors have had experience. Their application is therefore facilitated, particularly under conditions where bulky apparatus would render measurements difficult.

The Needles.—Ordinary hypodermic needles are employed with the phlebomanometer. For satisfactory results the needles, of course, should always be *clean and fully patent* before being used. The length should be

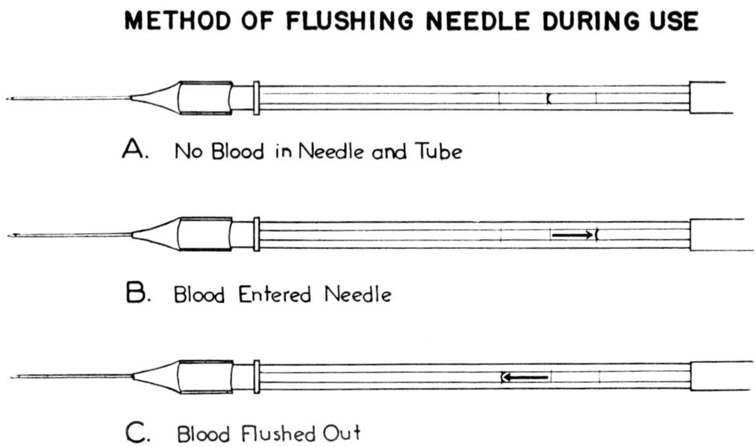

FIG. 98.—Schematic representation of method of determining whether or not the needle contains blood. For example, if at the time a venipuncture is made, the meniscus is at the middle transverse line shown in *A*, when the needle enters the vein, the venous pressure forces blood into the needle and the meniscus is moved to the more proximal transverse line shown in *B*. When the pressure in the manometer system is raised and the meniscus moves toward the needle and passes the original position before the puncture is made, *C*, then the observer knows that most of the blood has been flushed out of the needle. Such flushing of the needle with the citrate solution is important in preventing clotting and obstruction of the needle during more prolonged periods of observation.

$1\frac{1}{4}$ to $1\frac{1}{2}$ inches. The bore may be 23, 24, or 25 gauge. It is the narrow bore of the needle which prevents venous blood from rushing too rapidly into the observation tube before counterpressure can be established with the pressure bulb of the phlebomanometer. In subjects with high venous pressure, therefore, a 25 gauge needle should be employed, a 24 gauge for intermediate pressure levels, and a 23 gauge for normal or relatively low pressure. It is usually possible to predict the approximate level of pressure from the clinical study.

Since the measurements are made with the meniscus at a standstill and there is no friction to flow in the needle and observation tube, there being no flow of fluid, a small needle will not introduce an error in the determinations. Furthermore, a small, sharp needle causes little pain during the venipuncture. Also, because local damage to a vein is minimal, many determinations may be made in any given vein.

With the small needle, small veins may be entered in any part of the body where they can be seen, and measurements are not limited to large veins. Veins of the hands, feet, legs, abdomen, chest, face and viscera may be studied. Edematous areas may be transilluminated with an ordinary pocket flashlight, and the vein may be punctured deep in the tissues. If determinations of venous pressure are to be used to fullest advantage, measurements should be made anywhere necessary on the surface of the body, even internally during surgical procedures.

Method of Locating the Phlebostatic Axis and Phlebostatic Level.—The phlebostatic axis and level are located from the anatomic landmarks on the chest, as described previously (page 85). It is necessary to determine the relationship of the vein under study to the phlebostatic level. This is best accomplished by a spirit level mounted on a relatively long light strip of wood or aluminum rod. Other methods may be improvised to meet the particular situations of the observer.

It is better to bring the vein under study to the phlebostatic level whenever possible, as this eliminates the need for making corrections for the phlebostatic level (Fig. 99). This can be achieved easily when veins of the

POSITIONING OF VEIN TO PHLEBOSTATIC LEVEL

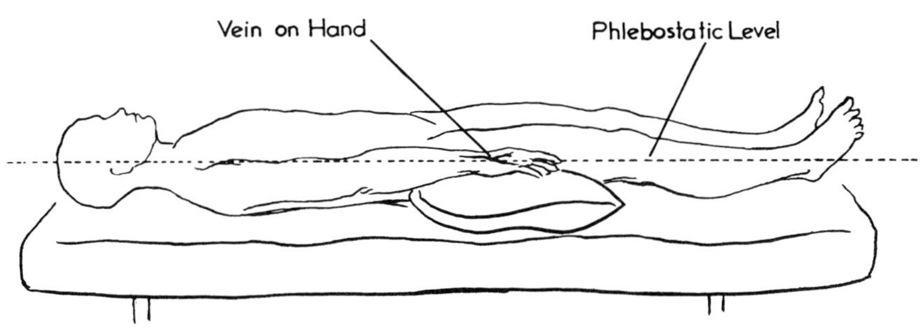

Fig. 99.—Whenever possible, the vein is brought to the phlebostatic level for measurement of venous pressure.

extremities are under study. When circumstances make it impossible to bring the vein to heart level or to the phlebostatic level, corrections for position or effects of gravity must be made. Correction for effects of gravity are made from measured distances of the vein under study above or below the phlebostatic level.

Corrections for Gravity.—*Corrections for gravitational effects when the vein is above the phlebostatic level* are made as shown in Figure 100. When the *vein is above the phlebostatic level,* the venous pressure is *decreased* by an amount in millimeters of water equivalent to the number of millimeters the vein is above the reference level. Corrections involving the specific gravity of the blood rather than that of water should be employed for highest accuracy. The resultant value indicates what the pressure would have been if the vein had been at the level of reference.

For example, in Figure 100 a vein of the abdomen is shown to be 50 mm. above the phlebostatic level. Therefore, the pressure obtained should be

CORRECTING FOR PHLEBOSTATIC LEVEL

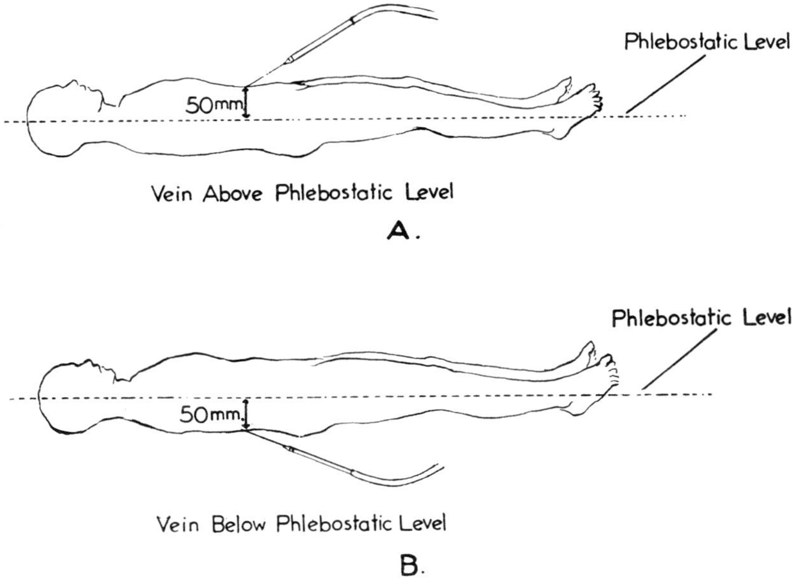

Fig. 100.—Method of correcting for position of vein to pressure at phlebostatic level. For example, if the vein is 50 mm. above the phlebostatic level, 50 mm. is added to the measured value of the manometer to obtain its value for the reference level. If the vein is 50 mm. below the phlebostatic level, 50 mm. must be subtracted from the measured value to obtain the pressure for the phlebostatic level or the level of reference.

increased by 50 mm. of water to obtain the pressure that would exist if the vein were at the phlebostatic level. If the *vein is below the phlebostatic level,* as in Figure 100 *B,* then the observed pressure in millimeters of water should be reduced by an amount equal to the distance in millimeters that the vein is below the phlebostatic level.

Influences of External Pressure.—When venous pressure is being measured, it is important to remove all constricting clothing or pressure-producing devices. These may obstruct flow of venous blood and produce an elevation in venous pressure, thus introducing an error through interference with venous return. Likewise, when the venous pressure is being measured in tissues pressed upon by the examining table, erroneous values will be obtained, since external pressure will be transmitted into the local veins (Fig. 101). It is well to keep in mind that errors may be produced when the position of the body is changed. For example, when the subject moves from the supine to the erect position, the shoulder, which naturally falls because of gravity, may compress the axillary or subclavian veins and produce elevations in pressure in distally located veins of the arm.

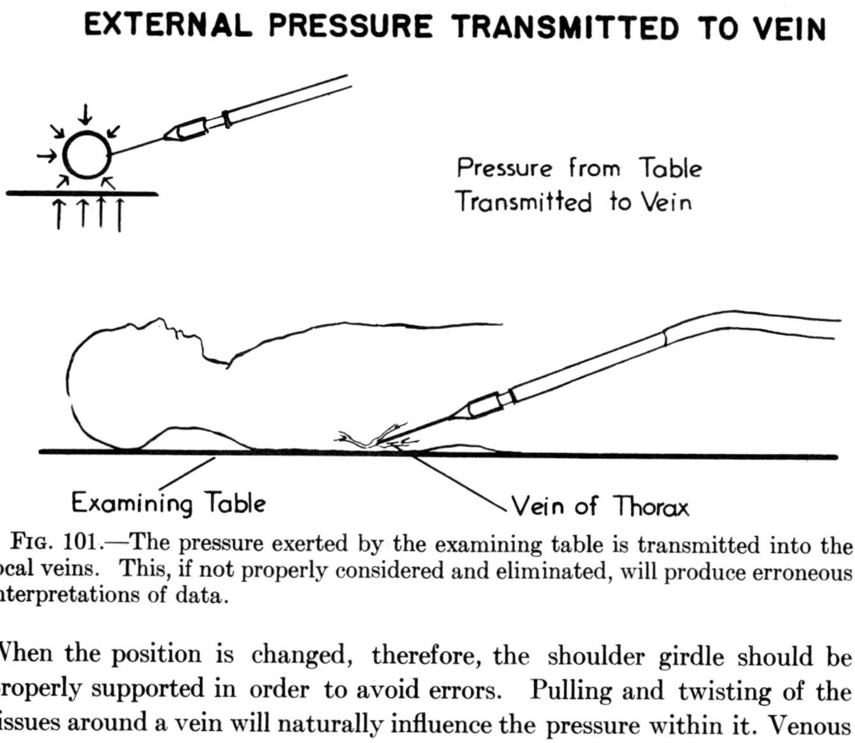

FIG. 101.—The pressure exerted by the examining table is transmitted into the local veins. This, if not properly considered and eliminated, will produce erroneous interpretations of data.

When the position is changed, therefore, the shoulder girdle should be properly supported in order to avoid errors. Pulling and twisting of the tissues around a vein will naturally influence the pressure within it. Venous pressure in parts being pressed upon, therefore, cannot be properly measured. The subject should be placed in such a position as to avoid these influences before the venous pressure is measured. These and other types of influences due to extrinsic pressure should be evident to the observer and should receive adequate consideration when measuring the pressure in a vein.

The Subject.—The subject should be relaxed physically and psychically, for the state of muscular contractions and the phase of respiration, as well as vascular tone, influence venous pressure. Relaxation can be satisfactorily achieved by proper approach to the subject. For best results he should be in the supine position on a firm, wide examining table covered with only a thin pad. He should be as nearly horizontal as possible; unfortunately, some ill subjects cannot rest comfortably in this position. Effects of position of the body and parts should always be borne in mind.

The subject should remain in the relaxed position for at least fifteen minutes before measurement of venous pressure is attempted, in order to allow the circulation and blood volume to achieve a new state of equilibrium of pressure and distribution of blood. A change in position introduces influences of gravity which will alter the circulation, especially that in the venous system. *When repeated measurements are made, the position of the body and part should be duplicated in every instance if the measurements are to be compared.*

Respiration should be free and easy. If there is dyspnea and labored breathing, the venous pressure will be altered accordingly (Chapter 2). It is also necessary to consider the influence which drugs, previous activity, meals, and other factors have on the state of veins and hemodynamics in general. Attention to such factors will avoid errors in comparison of serial data as well as in interpretation of results.

Venous Spasm.—When a vein is punctured with a needle, local trauma often produces constriction of the smooth muscle locally in the segment of vein. It is therefore advisable to allow three to five minutes to elapse before a final measurement is made (Fig. 102).

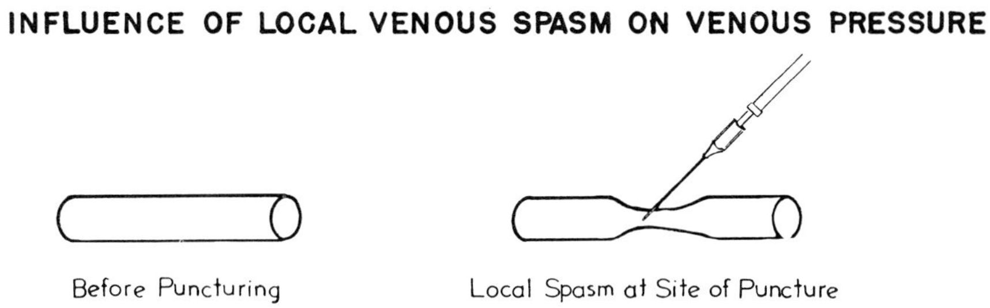

FIG. 102.—Venospasms produced locally by needle puncture. This will alter the venous pressure in the segment under study.

Furthermore, the psychic disturbance produced in the subject by the mere thought of a venipuncture and the sight of his physician, apparatus and needle, may produce generalized vasospasm and disturbances in venous pressure. Fortunately, the small needle and the relatively mild pain produce less disturbance and predispose to a rapid recovery of local venous spasm.

Sodium Citrate Solution.—A 2 per cent solution of sodium citrate in distilled water is isotonic and will inhibit clotting. This may be prepared sterile in a physician's office, laboratory or hospital. It is most convenient if placed in ampoules of 1 cc., a volume sufficient for many measurements. Ampoules of the solution may be purchased commercially.

Chapter 4

NORMAL VALUES OF VENOUS PRESSURE

Changes associated with varying conditions in normal and diseased subjects are of far greater importance than the average venous pressure. Unfortunately, measurements of venous pressure have been limited, primarily because of absence of a simple method of determination and also because of general lack of interest in the venous system among clinicians. With the advent of the syphgmomanometer interest was aroused mainly in arterial hypertension, and the venous system was neglected for many years. Because of its large size and ready accessibility, the median basilic, commonly and erroneously referred to as the antecubital, vein has been the most frequent site for measurement of venous pressure. In fact, with few exceptions, the normal values for venous pressure in man quoted in the medical literature are concerned almost exclusively with the median basilic vein, though there are obviously many clinical states which require measurements in other veins. It is hoped that the phlebomanometer, with its small needle and adaptability, will stimulate more extensive use in clinical medicine and research of determinations of venous pressure in as many other veins of the body as possible. Normal values for veins other than the veins of the antecubital areas possess limited value clinically because of the paucity of the studies.

The influence of age, sex, race, occupation, drugs, growth, and many other factors concerned with venous pressure in normal man has likewise been neglected. Obviously, disease states also deserve extensive study. It is, therefore, important to remember that the reported normal values of venous pressure are inadequate and do not include satisfactory evaluation of many variables.

When due consideration is given such factors as position of the subject, constricting clothing, pressure from external and internal sources, phlebostatic level, relaxation of the subject, state of respiration and other variables which influence venous pressure, the values shown in Figure 103 are essentially normal for the median basilic vein in the normal adult. The average pressure is 97 mm. of water, with extremes of 50 and 140 mm.

PRESSURE IN THE MEDIAN BASILIC VEIN

Right and Left Median Basilic Veins.—There is no significant difference in pressure in the right and left median basilic veins (Fig. 104). Some discrepancies may be noted from time to time because of the influence of

NORMAL VENOUS PRESSURE IN ADULT MAN

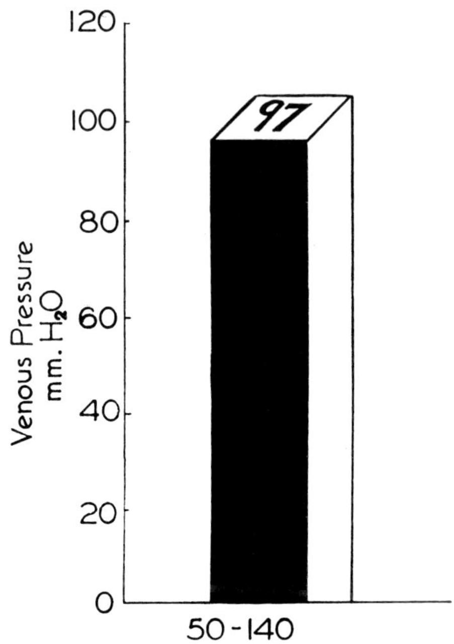

FIG. 103.—Average and extreme values of venous pressure in median basilic vein of normal adult man. In this illustration and all similar ones to follow, the mean value is indicated at the top of the column and the extremes near its base.

variables previously mentioned. Either or both veins may be used clinically. Differences between the pressures in homologous veins are due to well known mechanisms. The clinician or investigator should remember that differences may exist in a given individual, and a great many additional measurements will be required to ascertain their magnitude.

Sex.—There appears to be no clinically significant difference due to sex, although the venous pressure is 10 to 20 mm. of water lower in women than in men (Fig. 105). This tendency for males to have slightly higher pressure than females has been fairly well established for the basilic vein. Its clinical and physiologic significance must await more comprehensive analysis.

Race.—No significant difference in the venous pressure in the median basilic vein of normal white and Negro adults has been discovered (Fig. 106). Measurements in a large series of subjects of various races during health and disease are, of course, necessary before any final statement can be made.

BILATERAL VARIATION IN VENOUS PRESSURE – BASILIC VEIN

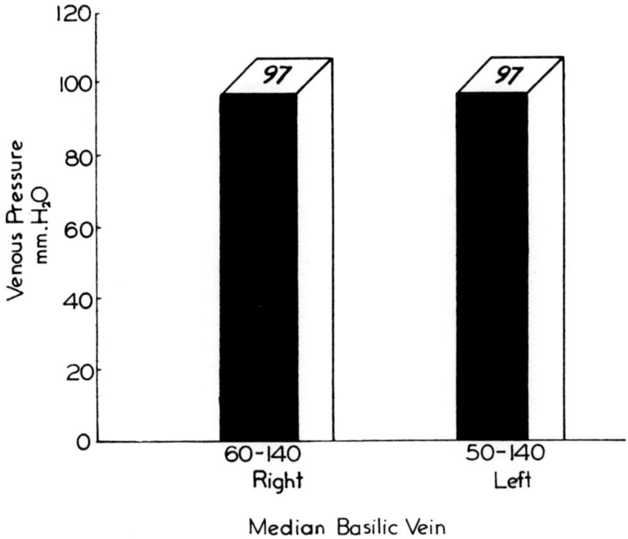

FIG. 104.—Venous pressure in the right and left median basilic veins of normal adults.

VARIATIONS IN VENOUS PRESSURE WITH SEX

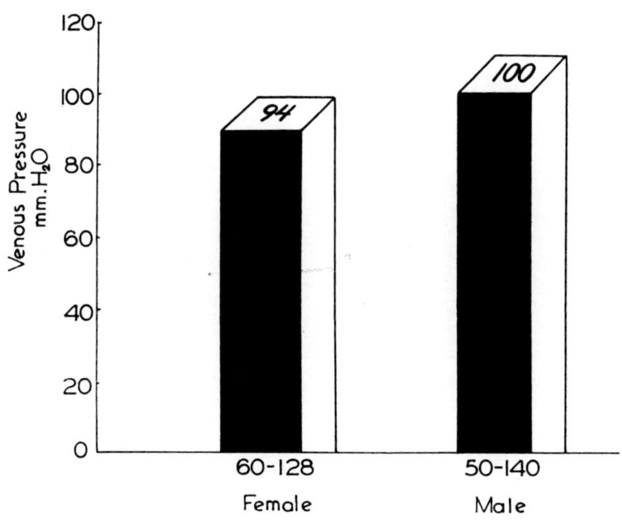

FIG. 105.—Variations with sex in normal venous pressure in the median basilic vein. The pressure tends to be slightly higher in males.

Age.—After adulthood venous pressure tends to decrease slightly with increasing age in normal man, although this factor has not received sufficient attention for accurate evaluation. The mean values for the median basilic vein in children of three to five years of age is about 46 mm. of water, with a range of about 30 and 63 mm. (Fig. 107). In children within the age

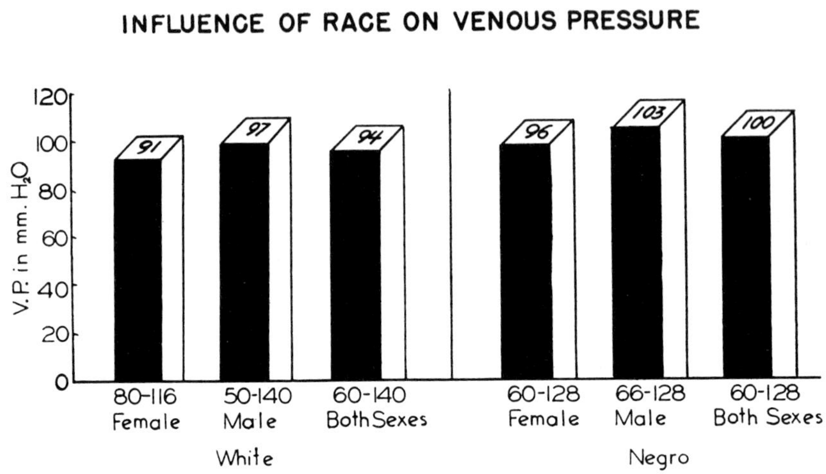

FIG. 106.—Venous pressure in the median basilic vein of normal white and Negro adults.

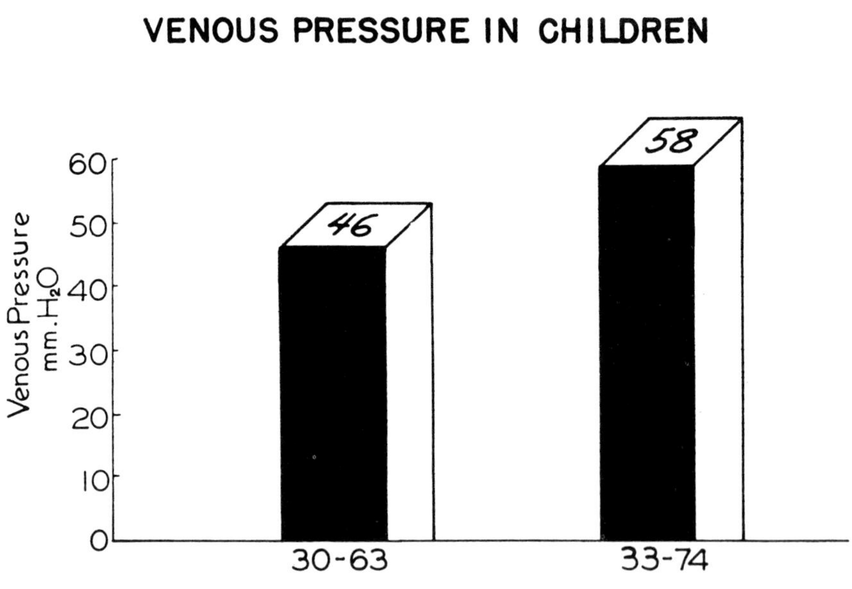

FIG. 107.—Venous pressure in the median basilic vein of normal children.

group of five to ten years venous pressure is slightly higher than in those of the younger age groups, the mean being 58 mm. and the extremes 33 and 74 mm. respectively (Fig. 107).

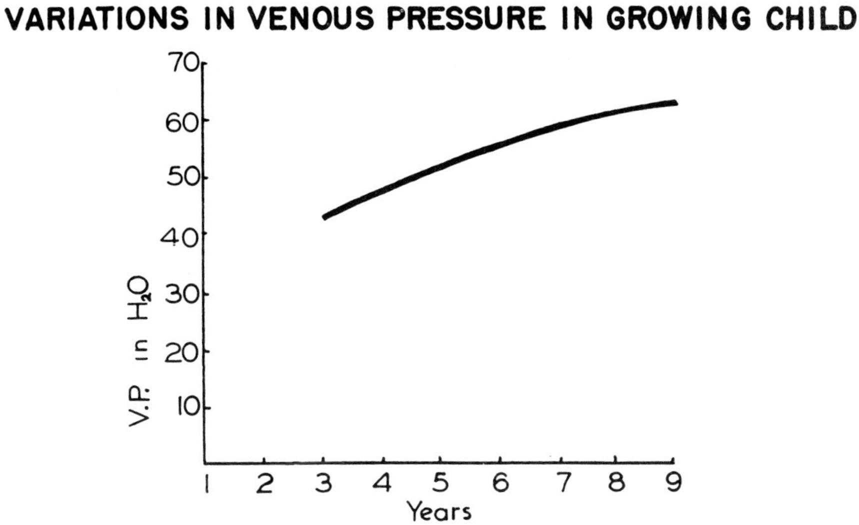

FIG. 108.—Trend of venous pressure in growing normal children.

The influence of age of children upon venous pressure in the median basilic veins is indicated graphically by Figure 108. Measurements in infants and adolescents are particularly deficient.

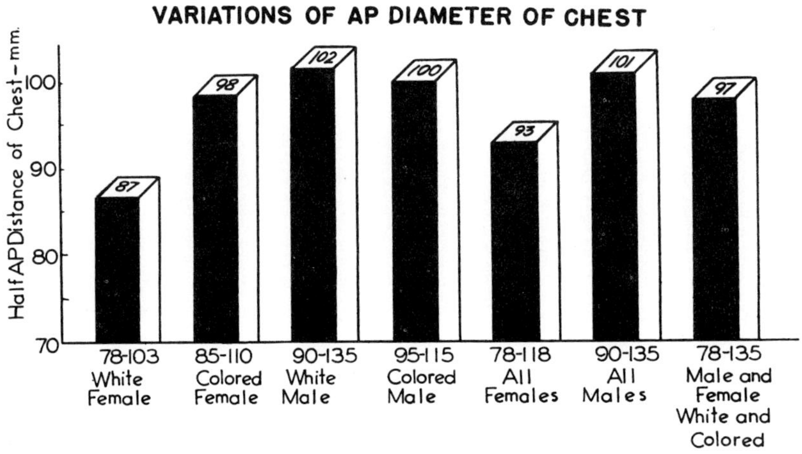

FIG. 109.—One-half the anteroposterior diameter of the chest of normal white and Negro adults. The wide variations in thickness of the chest are evident.

Influence of Anteroposterior Diameter of the Chest.—Since the anteroposterior diameter of the thorax varies considerably (Fig. 109), it is important to establish a level of reference for venous pressure which is not influenced unduly by variations in thoracic thickness. This has been discussed in greater detail in Chapter 2. It is further evident that the phlebostatic level is satisfactory as a reference level from Figure 110. From a practical clinical point of view, it is fortunate that the pressure in the median basilic vein is essentially the same in subjects with narrow and thick chests when measurements are referred to the phlebostatic level (Fig. 110).

RELATION OF THICKNESS OF CHEST TO VENOUS PRESSURE

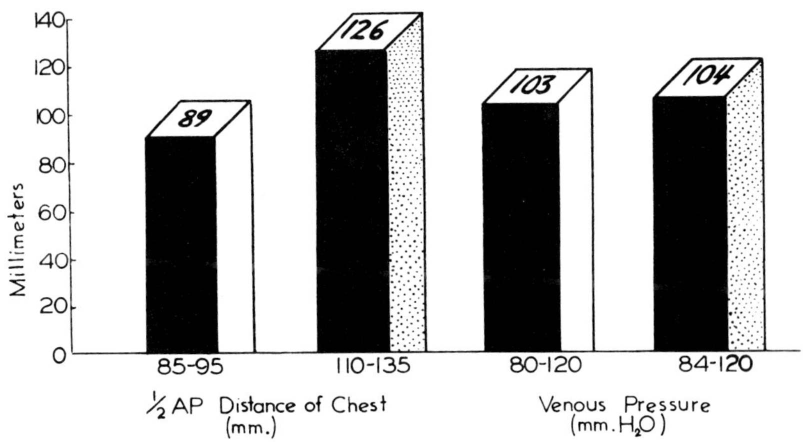

Fig. 110.—The venous pressure in the median basilic vein is essentially the same in subjects with short and long anteroposterior diameters of the chest if the phlebostatic level is employed as the level of reference or "heart level."

Influence of Direction of Needle on Pressure Recorded.—As indicated in Chapter 2, the direction of the beveled opening of the needle with respect to the direction of flow of the blood influences the pressure recorded. Higher pressures are recorded when the opening is directed against the direction of flow, and the more rapid the linear rate of venous blood flow, the greater will be the influence. Determinations should be made with the opening of the needle in the direction of the blood flow, unless there are special indications to the contrary.

PRESSURE IN VARIOUS OTHER VEINS OF MAN

Because of the need for measurements of pressure in veins other than the median basilic, inclusion of data here for various veins seems warranted, even though they are limited to a relatively small number of studies. Figure 111 summarizes some of the data for veins on the surface of the body of man, obtained from 100 normal adult subjects of both sexes and of the white and Negro races. Except under special circumstances, it is evident and, of course, consistent with hemodynamic principles (Chapter 2) that in general the farther the vein is from the heart, the higher will be the venous pressure.

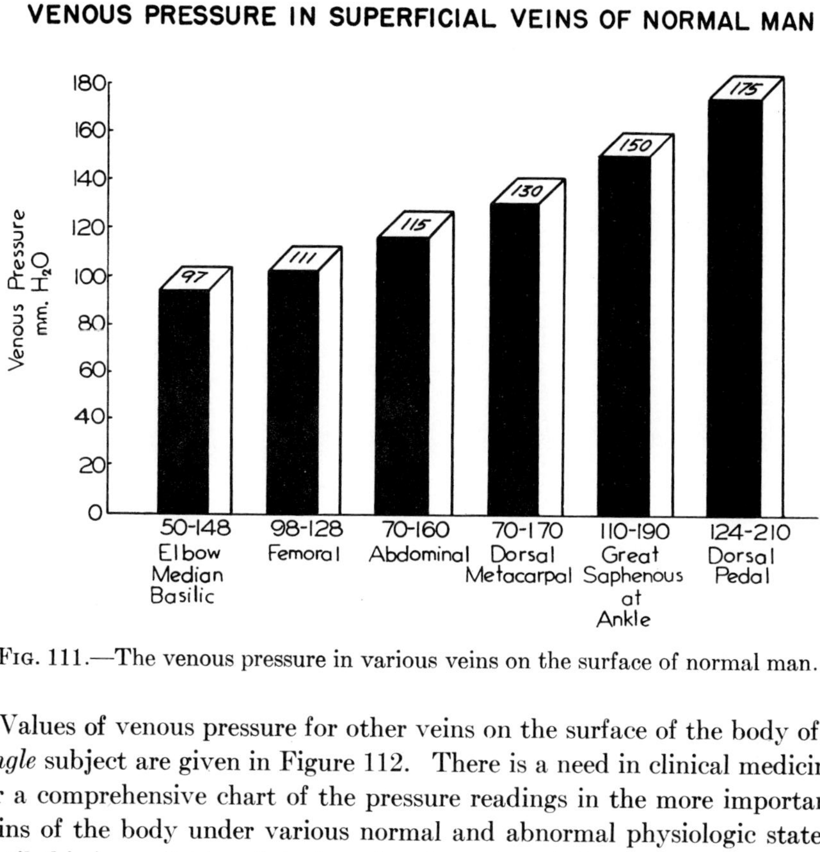

FIG. 111.—The venous pressure in various veins on the surface of normal man.

Values of venous pressure for other veins on the surface of the body of a *single* subject are given in Figure 112. There is a need in clinical medicine for a comprehensive chart of the pressure readings in the more important veins of the body under various normal and abnormal physiologic states. Until this is available, clinical applications of such determinations will remain restricted.

Portal Vein.—Venous pressure in the portal system of normal man has been reported to vary considerably. When the abdomen is opened, as in laparotomy, this pressure varies between 60 and 104 mm. of water; when closed, the range is from 150 to 220 mm. of water. Some observers consider 110 mm. to be definitely abnormal when the abdomen is open to the atmosphere. However, a much larger series of measurements will be necessary before any such definite statements can be considered valid.

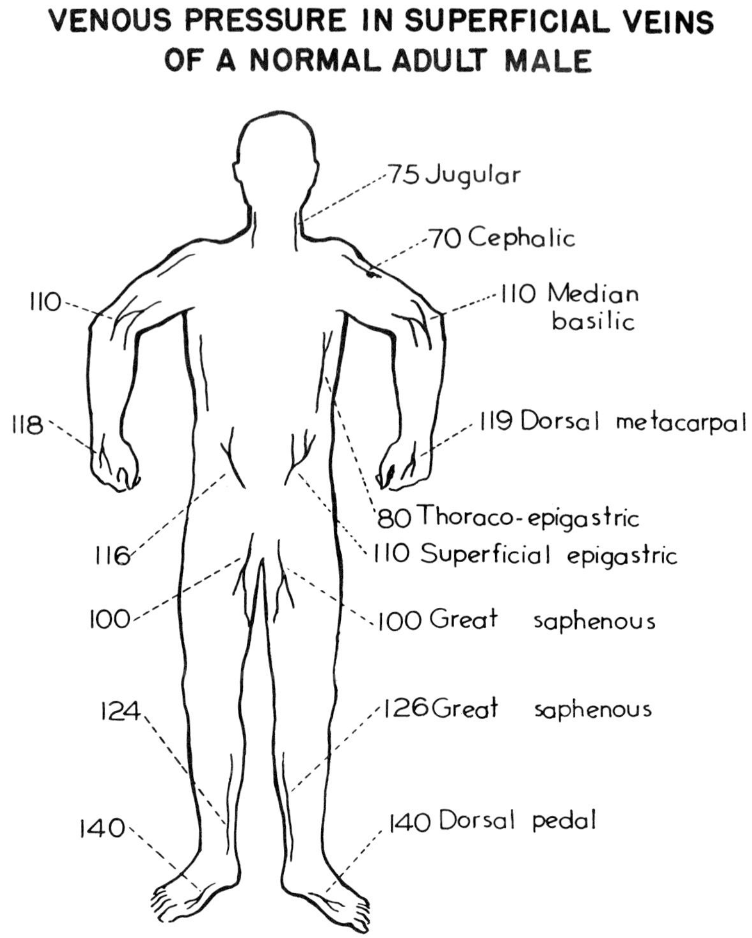

FIG. 112.—Diagram illustrating average venous pressure for superficial veins of normal man.

The advent of the venous catheter will initiate more extensive study of the deep veins of the body in intact man. With these data and others resulting from increased interest in venous pressure and therefore greater numbers of measurements, wider variations in values for normal and diseased man will be evident. It is hoped that all observers will find it possible to employ the same level of reference or "heart level," so that satisfactory comparison of data collected by various observers in different laboratories, clinics, and hospitals will be possible.

FACTORS VARYING VENOUS PRESSURE IN NORMAL MAN

For an appreciation of the measurements of venous pressure it is necessary to recognize the numerous factors which may influence these readings in diseased subjects as well as in normal man. The immediate discussions will be limited to factors which may vary the venous pressure in normal man and, of course, in subjects with disease as well. The disease states themselves, of course, may affect venous pressure even further. These will be presented in Chapter 5.

Gravity

As stated previously, the position of the vein of the body with respect to the phlebostatic level or "heart level" has an effect on the pressure in that particular vein. The method for reducing the value to a reference level has been discussed (Chapter 3). Obviously, when a man is standing, the force of gravity will tend to reduce the pressure in those veins which are above

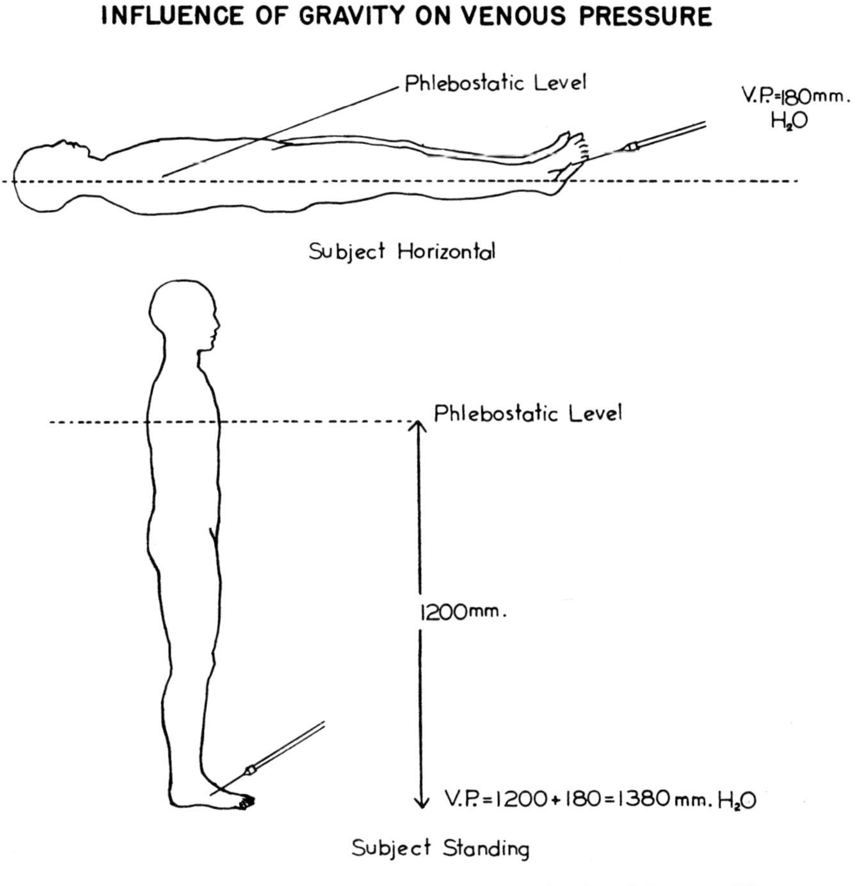

FIG. 113.—Venous pressure is influenced by gravitational forces. The venous pressure in a part below the phlebostatic level is equal to the venous pressure at the level of reference plus the gravitational force calculated from the distance of the vein below this level. Consult Chapter 3.

the phlebostatic level, *i. e.*, the veins of the shoulders, neck, and head, and to increase the pressure in the veins of the lower portions of the body. The greater the distance of the vein below the heart, the greater will be the elevation produced by gravity. In general, the degree of change in venous pressure produced by gravity is superimposed directly upon the pressure which would exist in the vein were it at the phlebostatic level (Fig. 113). Of course, this is true if such factors as muscular activity are not affecting venous return. When these factors are controlled, the effects of gravity will be found to behave in a predictable manner. Until more data are available, it is preferable to correct for position of the vein with respect to the phlebostatic level by the distance in millimeters between the vein and the level of reference.

Muscular Action

Venous valves cause muscular contractions to have a pumping action on blood flow. Henderson referred to this as part of the venopressor mechanism. The increase in intramuscular pressure with contraction of the muscle is transmitted into the vein coursing within and is imparted to the venous blood (Fig. 114). The pressure of the muscular tissue is readily transmitted

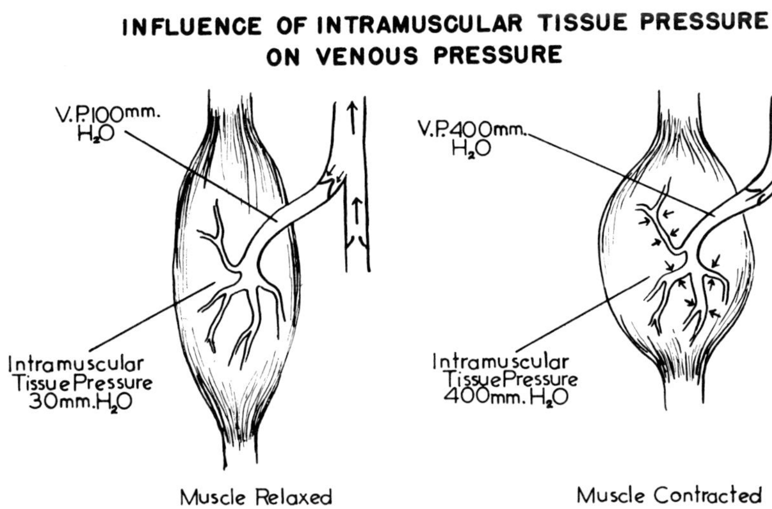

Fig. 114.—Intramuscular tissue pressure is relatively low when the muscle is relaxed but increases considerably when the muscle contracts, squeezing blood from the muscle into the extramuscular veins. This forces blood toward the heart.

to the blood within the veins because of their soft, pliable and collapsible walls. The more forceful the contraction of the muscle, the greater will be the elevation in pressure of the intramuscular tissue and, of course, the greater will be the elevation in pressure within the veins as well. As indicated previously (Chapter 2), because of competent venous valves blood is pumped toward the heart with each contraction.

It appears that maintenance of venous pressure, particularly when the subject is standing, is due in large part to the venopressor mechanism, including the influence of muscular tone or state of contraction upon venous pressure. Postural syncope is considered to be partially attributable to reduction in pressure of muscular tissue accompanying a decline in muscular tone. In disease or postinfectious states associated with myasthenia and syncopal episodes there is apparently a diminution in muscular tone and, in turn, pressure of muscular tissue. This effects a reduction in the venous pressure gradient and impairment in venous return when the subject is upright, and therefore syncope ensues.

If a subject is supine, exercise produced by successively lifting and lowering the right and left legs 10 times respectively elevates the venous pressure in the median basilic veins 20 to 50 mm. of water during the exercise (Fig. 115). This is probably consequent to an increased rate of

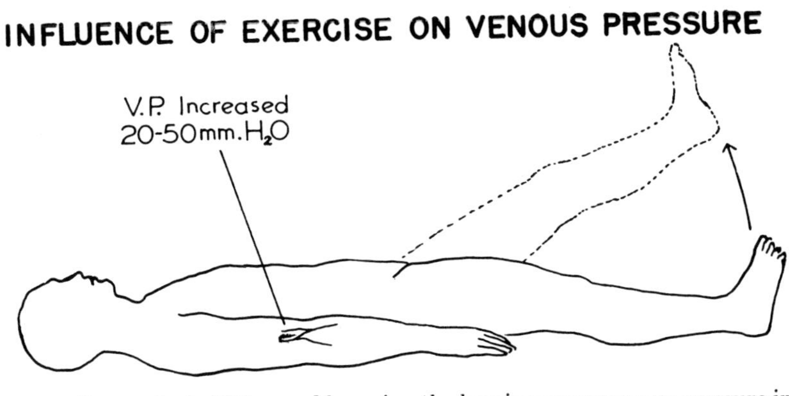

FIG. 115.—Successively lifting and lowering the legs increases venous pressure in the median basilic veins.

venous flow from the lower part of the body with greater filling of the veins near the heart and in the upper portions of the body. The venous pressure returns to its previous level about thirty seconds after the cessation of exercise. The action of exercise is further discussed in Chapter 5, where abnormal clinical states are presented.

Tissue Pressure

The pressure in other tissues besides muscle is transmitted to the blood in the veins coursing through them. It is necessary, however, to remember that the influence of tissue pressure upon venous pressure depends upon whether or not the change in the former is associated with (*a*) constriction or compression of the tissues or (*b*) expansion of the tissues.

a) **Increase in Tissue Pressure with Constriction and Compression of the Tissues.**—An example of this is muscular contraction, discussed in the preceding paragraphs and in Chapter 2. Other examples include contraction of fibrous tissue, as in scars or in certain disease states, such as scleroderma (Fig. 116). When the fibrous tissue contracts, the tissues in the

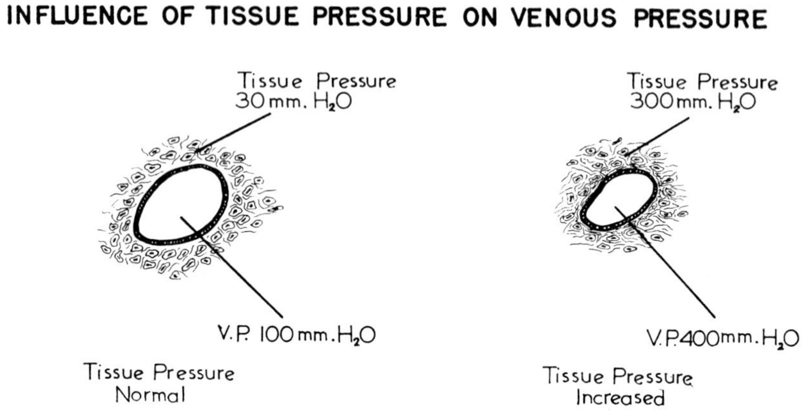

FIG. 116.—Venous pressure is increased in veins coursing through an area of diffuse contracting fibrous tissue.

surrounding area are "squeezed" together, with a resultant elevation in tissue pressure. This pressure is, in turn, imparted to the blood contained within the veins coursing through this area, and the venous pressure also rises.

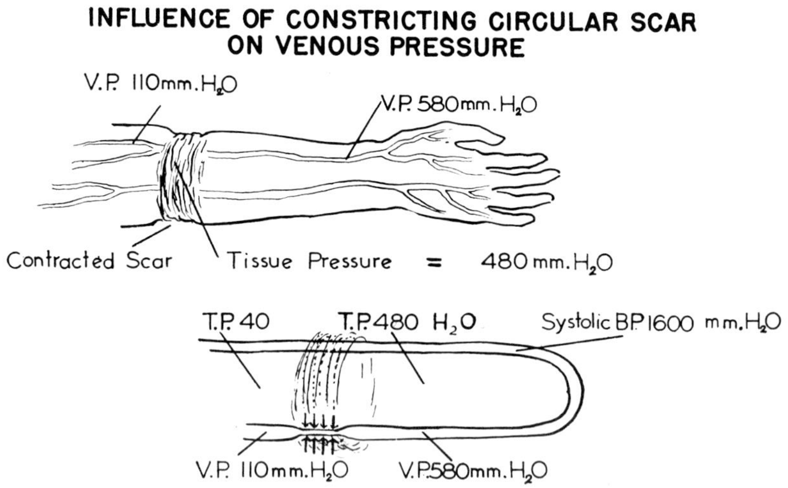

FIG. 117.—A local circular band of contracting fibrous tissue increases tissue pressure locally, obstructs venous flow, and increases venous pressure locally and distally in the vein and its tributaries. Consult the text for details.

Elevations in tissue pressure produced by constriction of the tissues create local disturbances in venous pressure, some of which are illustrated in Figures 117 and 118. A circular band of contracting fibrous tissue elevates the tissue pressure locally. This is transmitted not only to the veins within the constricting scar but also to the distal tributary veins (Fig. 117). The effect is analogous to the influence of a constricting cuff inflated to a pressure less than the systolic arterial blood pressure but above the diastolic blood pressure. The constricting cuff elevates the tissue pressure beneath the cuff and the pressure within the veins distal to the cuff. Since the pressure is higher beneath the cuff, venous flow ceases until enough blood has accumulated in the veins distal to the cuff to produce a pressure sufficient to overcome the pressure beneath the cuff, so that flow is re-established. The pressure transmitted from the arterial side of the circulation maintains increased venous pressure in the veins distal to the cuff, providing for a continual venous flow beneath the constricting cuff and venous return to the heart.

In the presence of diffuse constrictive fibrosis which includes the terminal portion of the circulation, such as exists in scleroderma of the hand and forearm, the venous pressure is elevated throughout the involved part (Fig. 118). Proximal to the involved portion the venous pressure drops to normal because of the normal tissue pressure (Fig. 118).

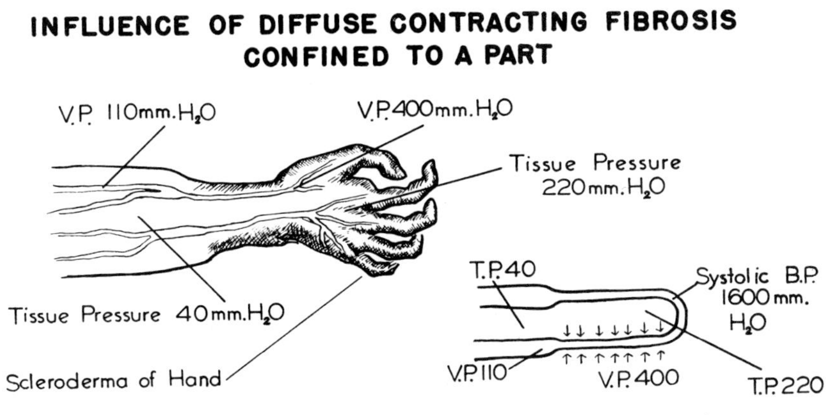

FIG. 118.—Diffusely placed contracting fibrous tissue increases tissue pressure locally and, in turn, increases venous pressure in the veins coursing within the involved areas.

b) **Increase in Tissue Pressure with Expansion of Tissues.**—An increase in tissue pressure in association with expansion of the tissues is best exemplified by edema within a part such as an arm (Fig. 119). When an arm becomes edematous, it expands and the skin is displaced away from the humerus and all tissues tend to be separated from each other. The fibrous trabeculae coursing through the part and attached to various structures within the part, including the walls of the veins, pull on the venous walls as the part expands, thus preventing the increased tissue pressure from effectively pressing upon the vein (Fig. 119). Because the hydrostatic pressure in the tissues is unable to press fully upon the vein, the increase in venous pressure tends to be less than would be expected in the absence of trabeculae.

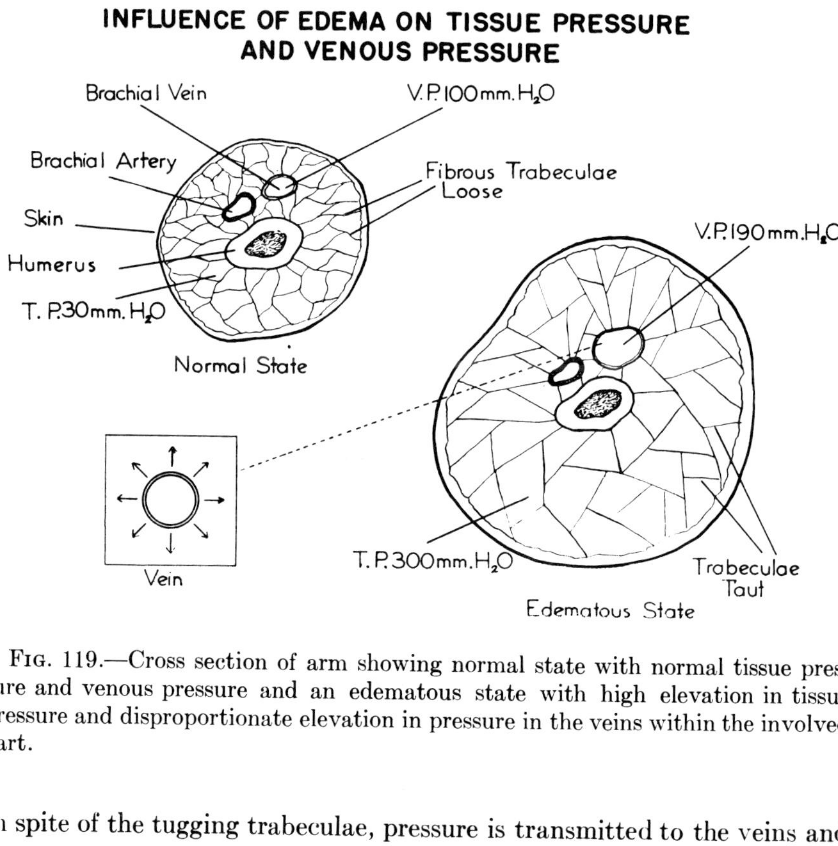

FIG. 119.—Cross section of arm showing normal state with normal tissue pressure and venous pressure and an edematous state with high elevation in tissue pressure and disproportionate elevation in pressure in the veins within the involved part.

In spite of the tugging trabeculae, pressure is transmitted to the veins and causes the venous pressure to be elevated. The blood volume in the venous system will influence the extent to which the tissue pressure is transmitted to the venous blood. The influence of trabeculae varies with veins, being more highly developed in small veins.

It is important to consider these types of actions of tissue pressure on venous pressure during interpretation of measurements obtained in veins coursing through tissues with abnormally high pressure. These factors may act either in a sharply localized area or generally.

Respiration

In the normal subject the effect of respiration upon venous pressure is increased as the thorax is approached. Pressure in the veins below the diaphragm tends to increase with inspiration, whereas that in veins which enter the thorax above the diaphragm decreases with inspiration. Expiration has an opposite action. The magnitude of the effects of respiration and the influence of various diseases, particularly of the chest and thoracic organs, requires considerable study in the clinic. Venous pressure should be recorded during quiet and relaxed breathing, when effects of respiration are minimal; otherwise, values may be obtained which are difficult to interpret or correlate with the clinical picture. Relaxation is important not only because of its influence upon respiration but also because of its effects on muscular tension.

When a recording is being made with the needle of the phlebomanometer in a vein in which respiration is having an effect, the meniscus will pulsate with the respiratory phases. It is customary to record the average venous pressure, or to have the subject *hold* his breath in mid-respiration for final balancing of the meniscus in the observation tube, or to record the value for the height of each phase of respiration. The latter determinations are usually of no clinical significance today because studies are lacking which would make their interpretation possible. As our knowledge of venous pressure increases, such measurements may have some clinical import.

Variations in pressure in the peripheral veins of man may be as great as 10 mm. of water during quiet breathing and are usually greater in athletes. The pumping effect of voluntary overventilation may produce a fall of 10 to 110 mm. of water in venous pressure (Fig. 120). Such a phenomenon would not exist during clinical measurements of venous pressure properly obtained. During defecation, micturition and parturition venous pressure is increased, as it is with the Valsalva experiment; all produce elevations in intrathoracic and intra-abdominal pressure. Quiet inspiration with mixed breathing increases the pressure 10 mm. in the lumen of the rectum, whereas inspiration during "pure" thoracic breathing is accompanied by a rise of 20 to 40 mm. of water. During the inspiration of "pure" abdominal breathing the rectal pressure rises 40 to 80 mm. of water, and coughing may be accompanied by an ascent of 180 mm. of water. Speaking produces an elevation of about 20 mm. of water. These fluctuations, reflecting changes in intra-abdominal pressure, have predictable influences upon the pressure of veins coursing through the abdomen. All the foregoing factors, as well as any concerned with a change in intra-abdominal pressure, such as tightness of the abdominal wall, presence of abdominal belts, state of the muscular tone and tension, must be considered when interpretations of measurements of venous pressure are made.

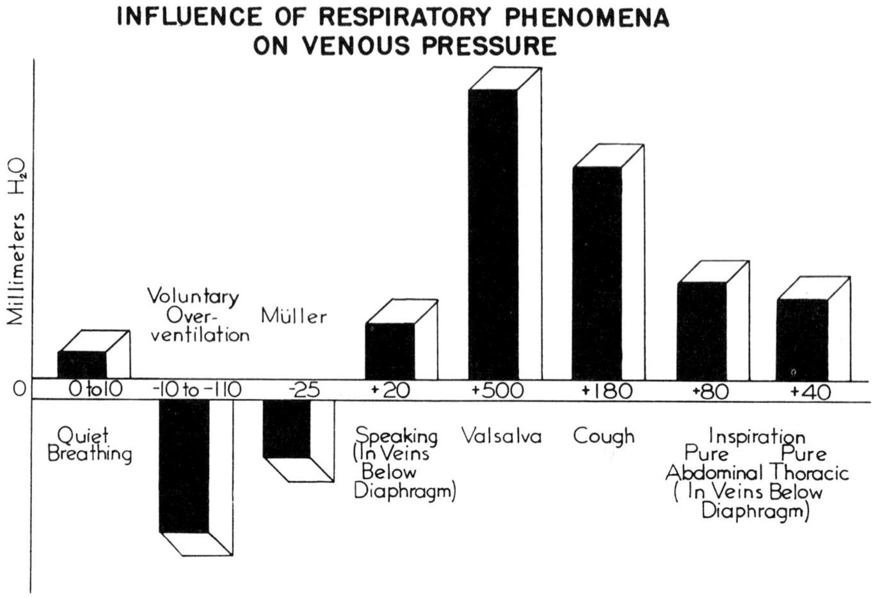

FIG. 120—Influence of respiration upon intraluminal pressure in the rectum and therefore upon pressure in the intra-abdominal veins of man as well as pressures measured directly in peripheral veins. This is a composite chart which indicates trends. Consult the text for details.

BED REST

Although the influence of prolonged periods of bed rest upon the venous pressure has not been adequately studied, it appears to exert a slightly depressive action.

SLEEP

Venous pressure tends to fall during sleep and to rise during the waking hours (Fig. 121). These diurnal variations are probably related to changes

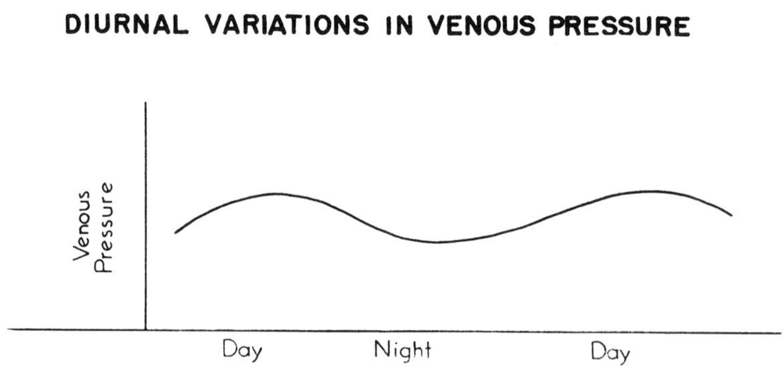

FIG. 121.—Diurnal variations in venous pressure.

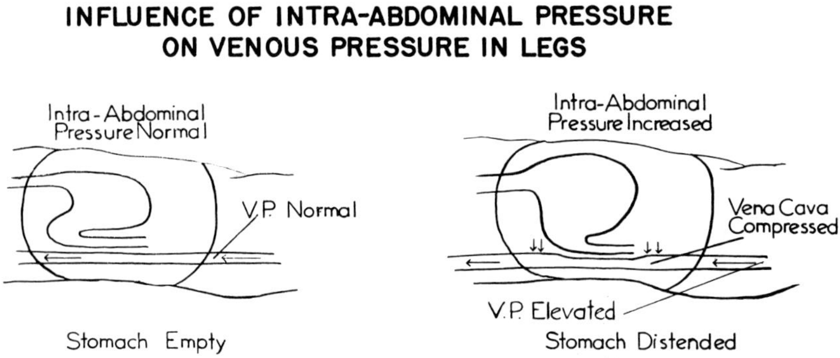

FIG. 122.—Intra-abdominal pressure is elevated by filling of the stomach with food and fluids. This increases pressure within veins whose blood courses through the abdomen.

in degree of muscular, respiratory, cardiac, neurogenic and psychogenic activity.

NUTRITION

Increase in intra-abdominal pressure with eating is at least partially responsible for the higher pressure in the veins coursing through the abdomen. The effect of food and water taken into the gastro-intestinal tract depends upon the volume of material introduced into the abdominal cavity and the increase in blood flow produced therein by digestion, as well as the looseness or tightness of the abdominal wall (Fig. 122). These and other factors associated with eating deserve more adequate evaluation.

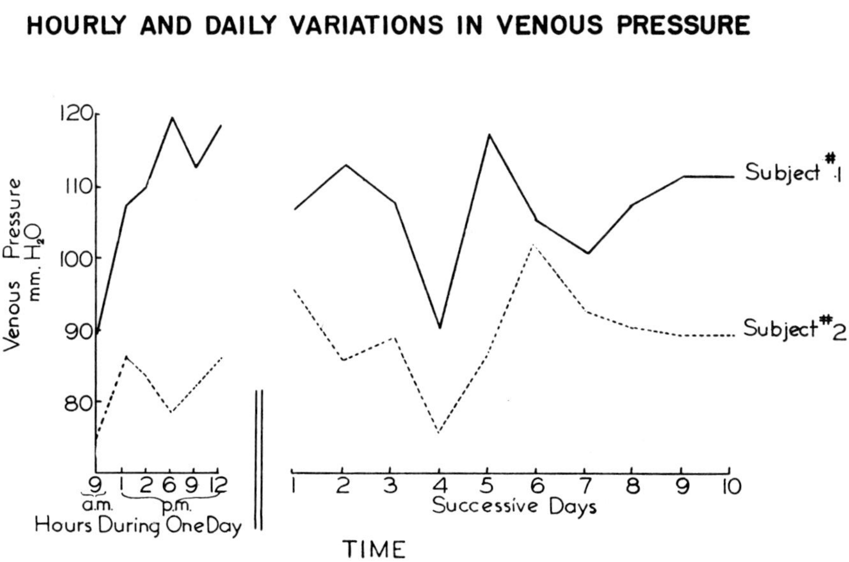

FIG. 123.—Hourly and daily variations in venous pressure in two normal subjects. (From Winsor and Burch, Am. Heart J., *31*, 387, 1946.)

Hourly and Daily Variations in Venous Pressure

Such variations have likewise not received extensive investigation, though they are of considerable consequence in proper evaluation of venous pressure, particularly when only slight changes are noted. Fluctuations are shown for two subjects in Figure 123.

Drugs

Drugs which affect the vascular system, particularly the veins, may alter venous pressure. Vasoconstrictor drugs, such as *epinephrine* and possibly nor-epinephrine, in proper amounts, will constrict the veins and raise venous pressure, whereas sympatholytic agents may lower it. *Nitrites* induce dilatation of the peripheral vessels, including the venules, and may reduce the level of venous pressure. It is not possible to enter into a discussion of all the various chemical agents which may modify the level of venous pressure, but their possible influence should always be considered in interpretations of the recordings.

Intravenous Administration of Fluids

Rapid intravenous administration of fluid is accompanied by an elevation in venous pressure, due to distention of the veins by the increase in blood volume. Fluids which are more effective in producing an increase in blood volume, such as plasma, whole blood, or solutions of gum acacia, are more apt to raise venous pressure (Fig. 124). Because the veins are so distensible,

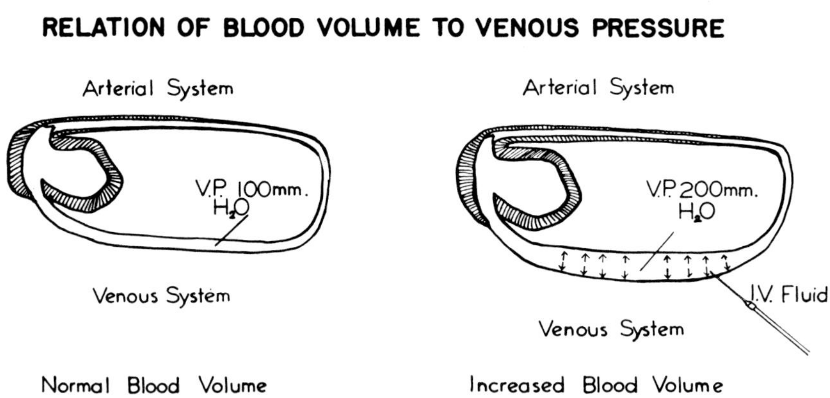

FIG. 124.—Factors which increase blood volume or reduce volume of the venous system tend to increase venous pressure. The former occurs from rapid intravenous administration of fluids.

they can accommodate a relatively large volume of fluid with relatively little change in venous pressure. Although fluids are administered in shock to increase the effective blood volume and to raise the depressed arterial and venous pressures, they may produce a deleterious elevation if injudiciously employed in disease states already associated with abnormally high blood volumes.

When the blood volume is increased, the additional blood accumulates mainly in the venous side of the vascular system, since the latter is more easily distended and has a lower pressure (Fig. 125). Fluid tends to accumulate in those portions of a continuous fluid system in which the pressure is lowest and in which the volume may be accommodated with the least change in pressure (Fig. 125).

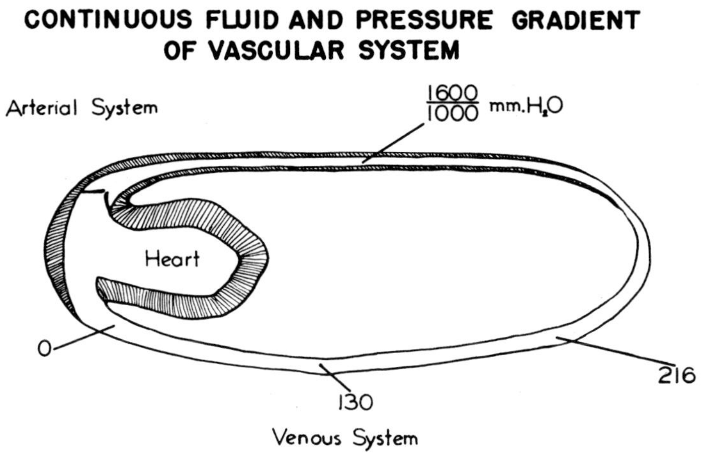

FIG. 125.—Diagram of continuous fluid system of the circulation. The pressure is highest in the relatively rigid arteries and lowest in the soft, pliable and easily distensible veins. Fluid administered will tend to accumulate in the veins.

Fluids freely diffusible through the capillary epithelium, such as physiologic solution of sodium chloride, increase the volume not only of the blood but also of all extracellular fluid. The former is increased more or less in proportion to the increase in interstitial volume. Ingestion of large quantities of sodium chloride intensifies hydration, with consequent increase in all extracellular fluid, including plasma volume and, therefore, in venous pressure.

BREATHING AIR ABOVE AND BELOW ATMOSPHERIC PRESSURE

When the pressure of the air breathed is above that of the atmosphere, venous pressure tends to rise and when it is below that of the atmosphere, within limits, venous pressure tends to fall (Fig. 126). The principal effect of the pressure of the air respired occurs indirectly through its influence upon the intrathoracic pressure.

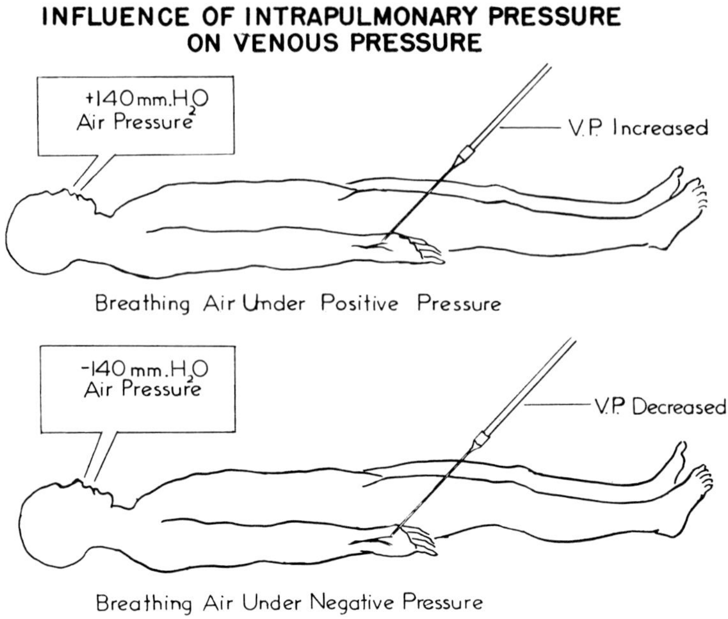

FIG. 126.—Influence of pressure of air respired upon systemic venous pressure.

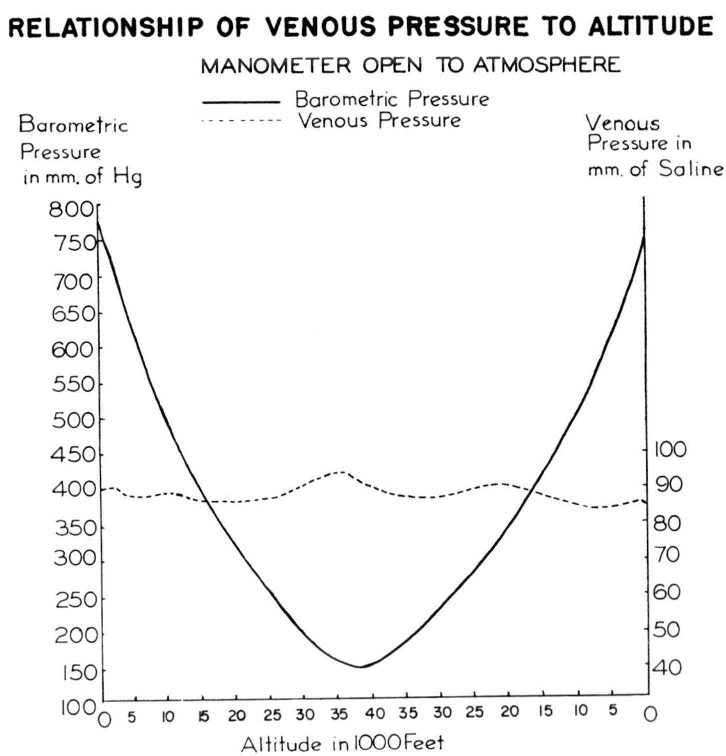

FIG. 127.—The venous pressure does not change, that is, it is essentially the same value above atmospheric pressure even with considerable change in the latter. Since the pressures were measured with the manometers opened to the atmosphere, the venous pressure was compared with that in the atmosphere. (Courtesy of Sutherland, Molumut and Brookes, J. Aviation Med., *14*, 280, 1943.)

Altitude

Altitudes up to 4000 feet produce little change in venous pressure, and there may be none with even much higher altitudes, provided they are reached slowly so that the influences of changes in barometric pressure may be reflected within the tissues and also provided no important physiologic changes occur because of deficient oxygen. However, sudden alterations in environmental pressure, such as may be created by sudden ascent or descent of aircraft or particularly under experimental conditions in pressure chambers, will affect the venous pressure. Figures 127 and 128 illustrate some of these effects when the changes in pressure occurred slowly and the venous pressure was measured in a closed and an opened system with the subjects in a decompression chamber.

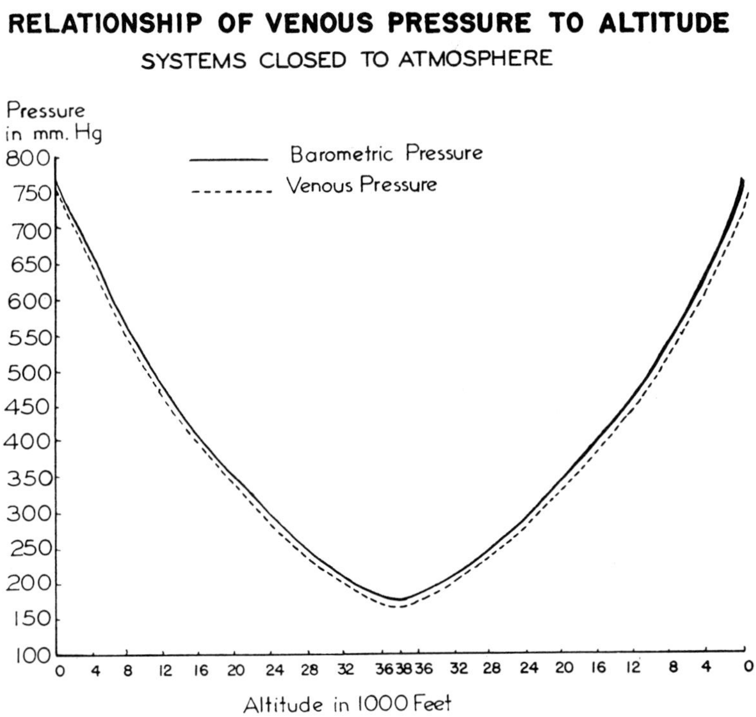

Fig. 128.—The absolute pressure in the venous system declines parallel to the decline in atmospheric pressure. This change in pressures or "absolute" pressures was measured with the manometers closed from the atmosphere. (Courtesy of Sutherland, Molumut and Brookes, J. Aviation Med., *14*, 280, 1943.)

Chapter 5

THE VENOUS PRESSURE IN CERTAIN ABNORMAL CLINICAL STATES

The influences of disease states upon venous pressure and, in turn, the clinical utilization of related pressure values to facilitate the understanding, diagnosis, and management of the respective diseases cannot be overemphasized. The physiologist and clinical investigator have long been aware of the importance of such determinations in clinical medicine. In spite of this, the clinician has neglected their use in the managment of his patients. Obviously, routine measurements of venous pressure are not to be advocated at this time, especially since they necessitate venipuncture, but certainly they should be obtained in clinical states in which they would provide valuable information. In most instances failure to take advantage of such determinations stems from a lack of adequate appreciation of their applicability. Although it is not possible to enter into a detailed discussion of the applications here, the presentations to follow are intended to indicate the general principles concerned with clinical measurement of venous pressure. It is hoped that with some imagination and correlation of anatomic, physiologic, and pathologic factors and the peculiarities of disease states the clinician will understand the broader and more general applications of these determinations.

VENOUS OBSTRUCTION

Lesions which produce an obstruction of a vein tend to result in elevation in the pressure in that vein and its tributaries distal to the obstruction

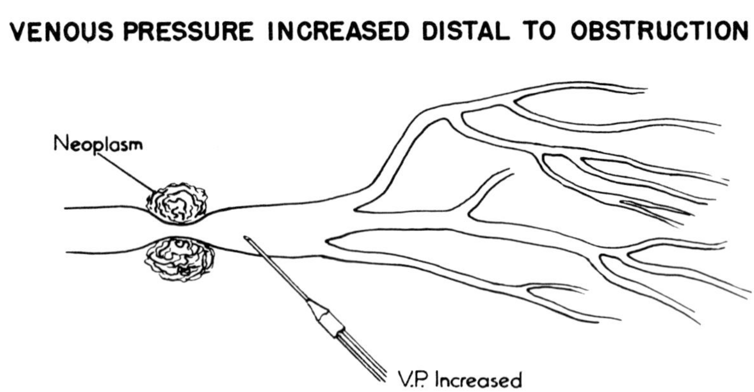

Fig. 129.—The venous pressure is elevated distal to a venous obstruction produced by a growing neoplasm.

(Fig. 129). If there is adequate collateral circulation, the venous pressure will remain essentially unchanged (Fig. 130). This is particularly true where there is an extensive network of veins, such as on the dorsum of the hand; the intercommunicating vessels permit adequate collateral circulation, so that an obstruction to one of the veins occasions only a negligible, if any, elevation of the venous pressure distally (Fig. 130).

VENOUS OBSTRUCTION WITHOUT INCREASE IN VENOUS PRESSURE

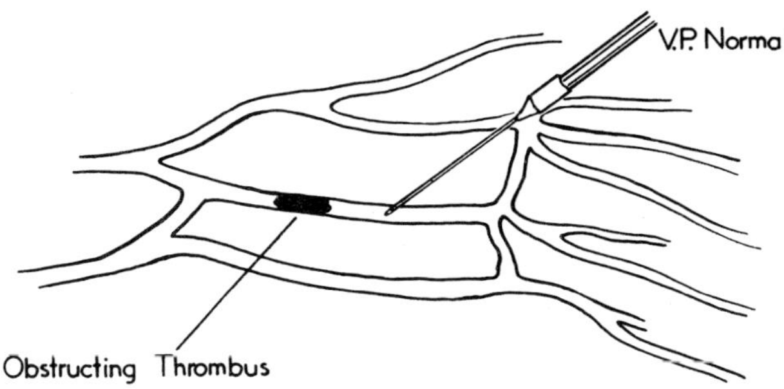

FIG. 130.—Network of veins on the dorsum of the hand. An obstructive lesion in a vein produces little, if any, elevation of pressure in the vein distally because of the extensive network of intercommunicating vessels permitting collateral circulation.

Obstruction to Main Venous Channels.—When the main venous channels are obstructed, the venous pressure in the distal portion of the vein and its tributaries is usually greatly elevated (Fig. 131). Since venous obstruction favors the formation of edema, the part drained by an obstructed vein is often edematous. Thus, measurement of the pressure in a vein or its tributaries will not only indicate obstruction but may also reveal a possible cause for any existent edema. In fact, in most clinical states with edema

VENOUS HYPERTENSION IN TRIBUTARIES OF LARGE VEINS

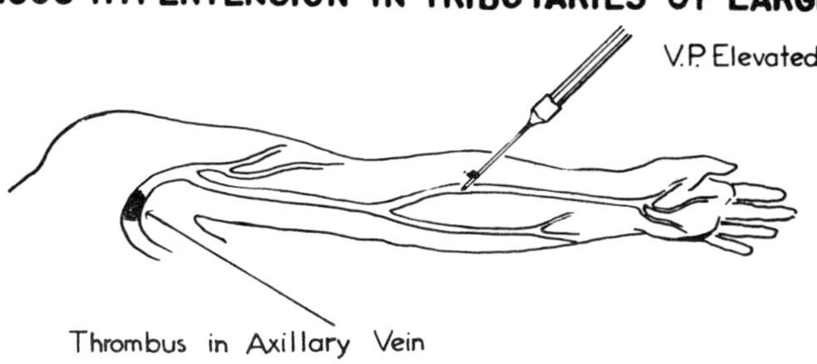

FIG. 131.—Obstruction of the axillary vein by a thrombus resulting in venous hypertension in veins of the arm.

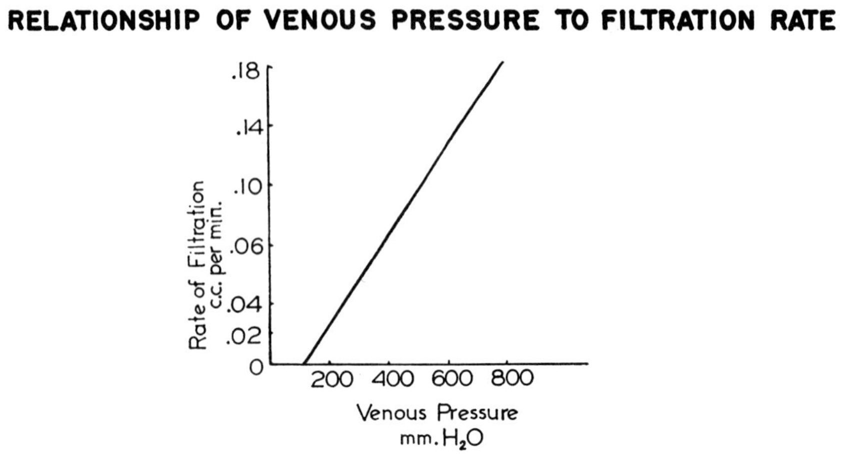

FIG. 132.—Diagram of the relationship of venous pressure to the rate of filtration of fluid from the blood vessels into the intercellular spaces. (Modified from Landis and Gibbons, J. Clin. Investigation, *12*, 117, 1933.)

comparison of measurements of venous pressure within the edematous area with those in the nonedematous areas will often aid considerably in clinical diagnosis. An elevation in venous pressure will produce an increase in the amount of intercellular fluid (Fig. 132) and edema, if other compensatory mechanisms are not adequate.

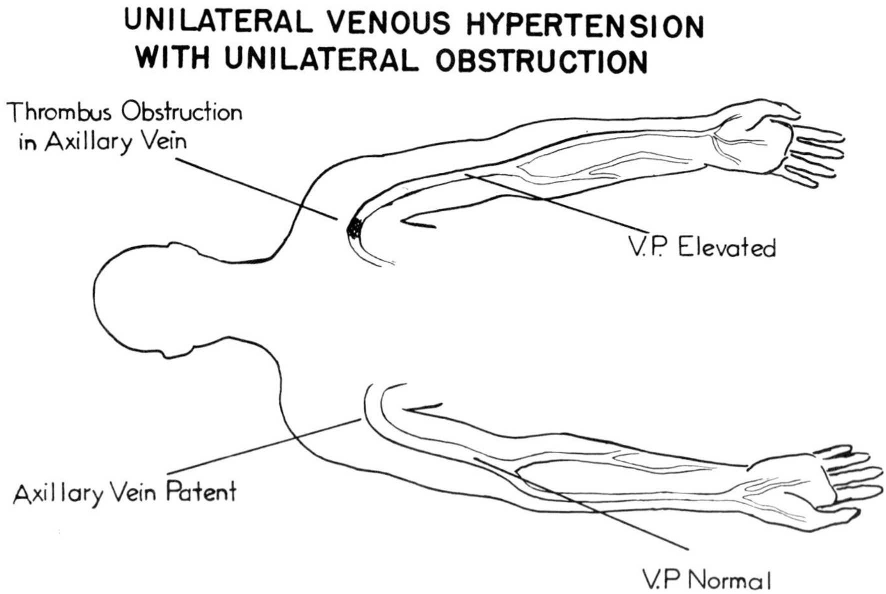

FIG. 133.—Venous hypertension present in veins of arm with obstruction to the axillary vein but not in those of the other arm with a patent axillary vein.

Measurement of venous pressure will also aid in excluding states which are accompanied by generalized venous hypertension. Since right ventricular congestive heart failure, for example, is associated with venous hypertension in all systemic veins, it will be excluded as a cause if comparison of the pressure in various veins reveals venous hypertension to be localized. Thus, if venous hypertension is suspected in the veins of an arm, due to obstruction to the axillary vein of that arm, it is important to measure the pressure in the veins of the other arm also (Fig. 133). The pressure in the tributaries of the obstructed vein will be elevated, whereas that in the contralateral veins without obstruction will be normal.

Localization of Venous Obstruction.—It is possible not only to detect the existence of venous obstruction but also to localize the obstruction sharply. For example, if the pressure is elevated in the veins of the arms, head, neck and chest above the level of the diaphragm, then the obstruction must be in the superior vena cava (Fig. 134). At the same time the venous pressure

OBSTRUCTION TO SUPERIOR VENA CAVA

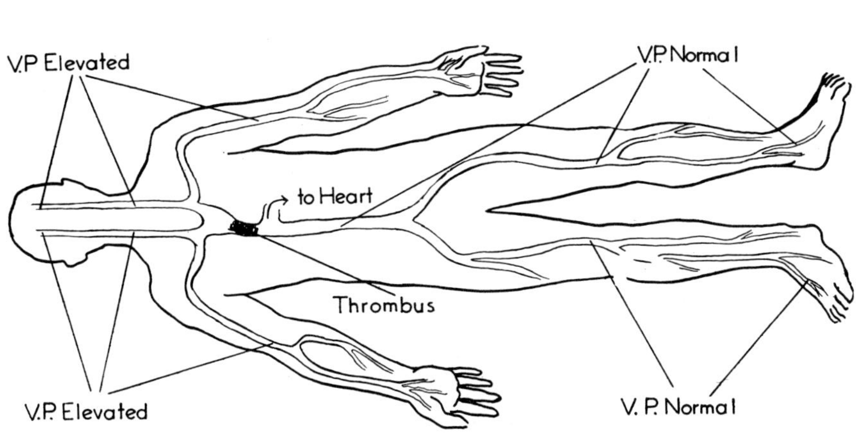

FIG. 134.—Obstruction to superior vena cava, producing venous hypertension above the level of the diaphragm and in the arms; pressure in the veins of the legs is normal.

in the tributaries of the inferior vena cava will be normal and it will be moderately elevated bilaterally in the inferior epigastric veins because of collateral circulation.

With obstruction to the superior vena cava it is possible to demonstrate reversal of direction of flow in the veins of the anterior thoracic wall (Fig. 135). When the superior vena cava is normally patent and the pressure in

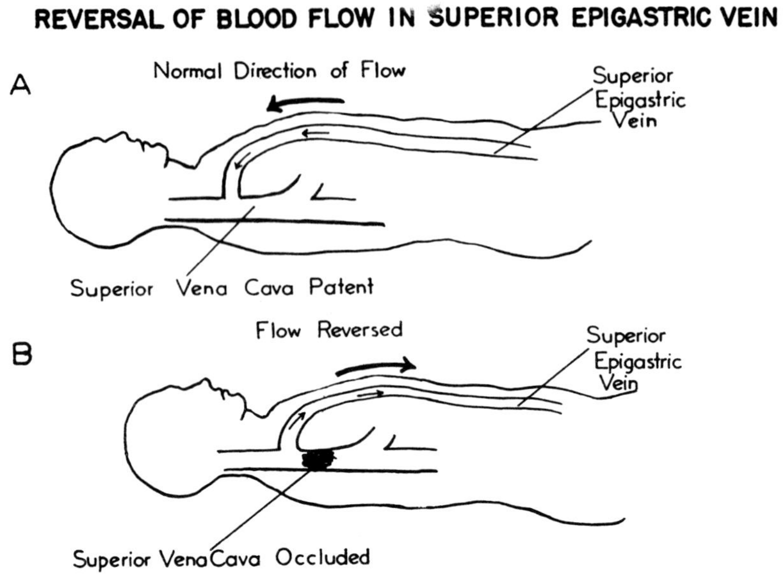

FIG. 135.—*A*, Normal cephalad direction of flow in the veins on the anterior surface of the chest with normal patency of the superior vena cava and, *B*, reversal of flow, caudad direction of flow, in the veins of the chest with obstruction to the superior vena cava.

the veins of the upper portion of the chest is normal, the direction of blood flow is cephalad when the subject is supine. When the superior vena cava is obstructed, the pressure is elevated in the veins of the chest and the direction of blood flow is caudad, that is, the flow is through the collateral venous system into the patent inferior vena cava and back to the heart.

Clinical Method of Determining Direction of Blood Flow in Veins.—The direction of blood flow is often of considerable value for better appreciation of measurements of venous pressure and recognition of the nature of the underlying disease. This is usually not difficult to determine in the veins of the body that are accessible for examination. A segment of the vein free from tributaries is selected for study. At one end of the venous segment pressure is applied with the tip of one index finger to occlude the vein immediately beneath the fingertip (Fig. 136). The tip of the other index finger is placed immediately adjacent to the one already occluding the vein and pressure is applied to occlude the vein beneath this second index fingertip also. The tip of the second index finger is then drawn with continued pressure along the length of the venous segment to "milk" it empty. If there aıe no tributaries entering the venous segment from the deep tissues, the segment will remain empty as long as the two ends of the segment are occluded by the fingertips. One finger is then lifted to release the local

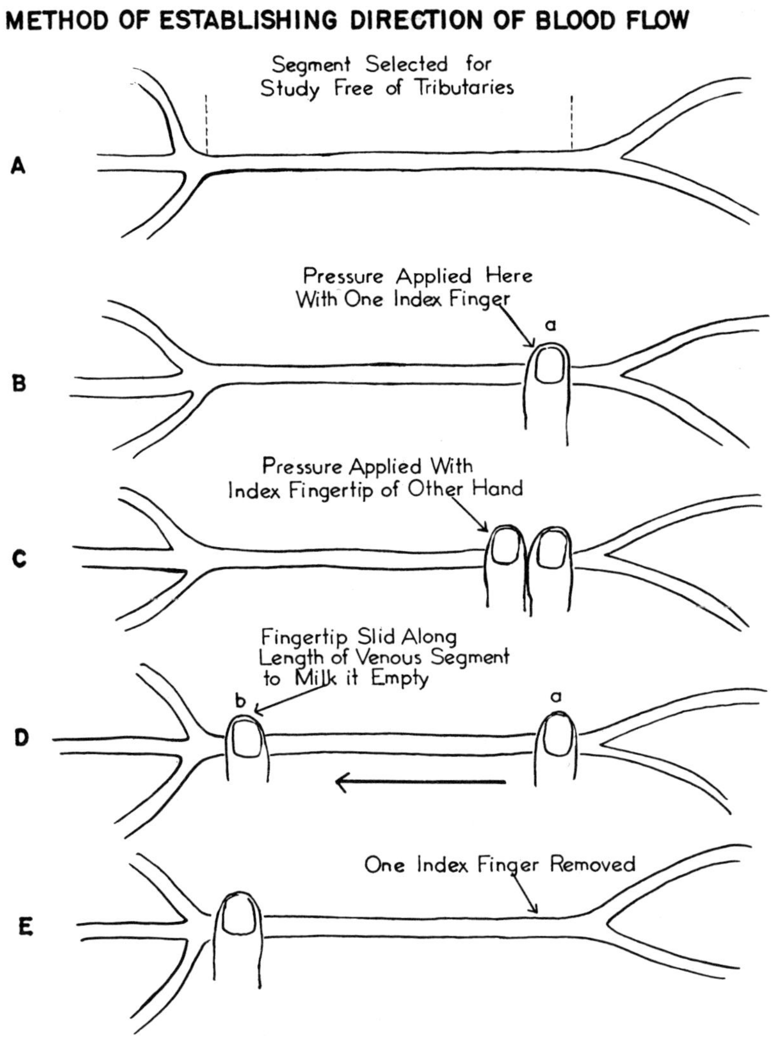

FIG. 136.—Diagrams show method for selecting, "milking," and establishing the direction of blood flow in a venous segment. Consult text for details.

occlusion, and the rate of filling of the venous segment is noted. The venous segment is again milked empty, the occlusion of the other end is released by lifting the other fingertip, and the rate of filling of the segment from this end is noted. This procedure is repeated until the observer has determined with certainty from which end the segment fills more rapidly. *Since the blood flows from the end which fills more rapidly to the end which fills more slowly, the direction of blood flow in the venous segment is thus established.*

Essentially the same procedure may be employed to determine the adequacy of function of venous valves (Fig. 137). The venous segment is selected and tributaries entering into the segment are occluded by pressure with a fingertip. Pressure is applied with a fingertip at the proximal end and the finger is slid to the other end in a direction opposite to that of the blood flow, where the digital pressure is maintained to occlude the distal end of the segment. This movement of the fingertip with pressure along the length of the venous segment "milks" it of blood. If there is an adequately functioning valve near the proximal end of the venous segment, the segment will remain empty. Proximal to the point of location of the venous valve the vein is distended with blood, whereas on the distal side it is empty. This may be tested satisfactorily with filled veins of the dorsum of the hand (Fig. 137). When there is a valve at both ends of the segment,

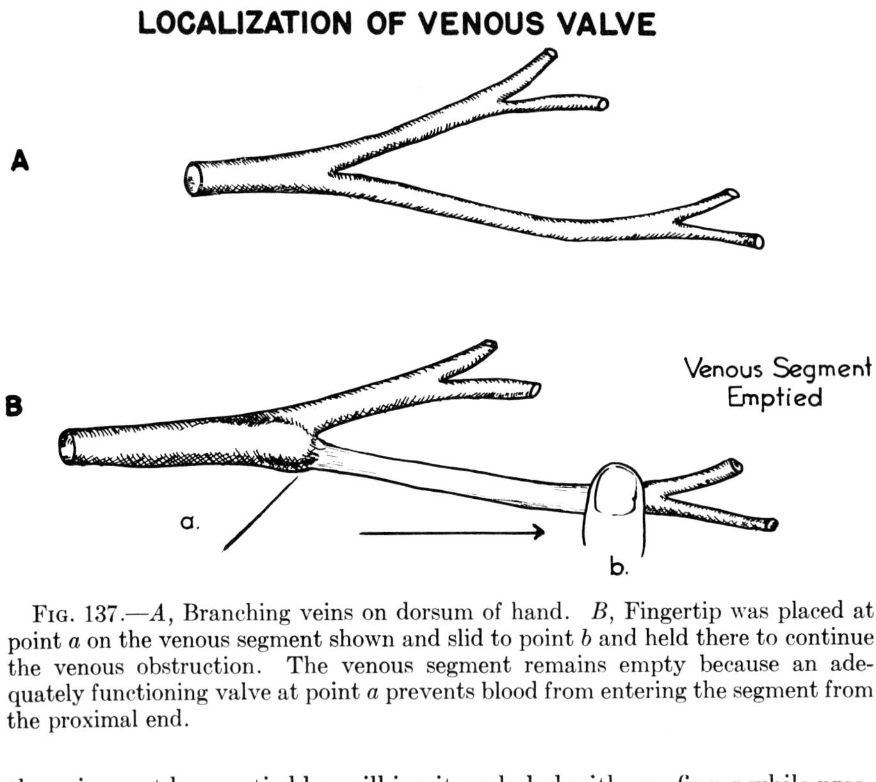

FIG. 137.—*A*, Branching veins on dorsum of hand. *B*, Fingertip was placed at point *a* on the venous segment shown and slid to point *b* and held there to continue the venous obstruction. The venous segment remains empty because an adequately functioning valve at point *a* prevents blood from entering the segment from the proximal end.

the vein must be emptied by milking it cephalad with one finger while pressure is maintained on the distal end with another finger, as shown in Figure 136.

Obstruction to Specific Veins.—As stated previously, obstruction to veins results in venous hypertension in the distal portion of the vein and its tributaries. Therefore, it is important for the observer to be familiar with the anatomy of the venous system in question, so that comparisons of venous pressure may be made with that of the contralateral veins. It is not possible in this type of presentation, nor is it necessary, to discuss obstruction to each of the main venous channels of the human body; only a few of the main ones will be treated.

a) *The Inferior Vena Cava.*—Obstruction to the inferior vena cava below the renal veins produces venous hypertension *only* in its tributaries, the veins of the legs and those of the lower abdominal areas (Fig. 138). The direction of blood flow in the inferior epigastric veins of the abdominal wall

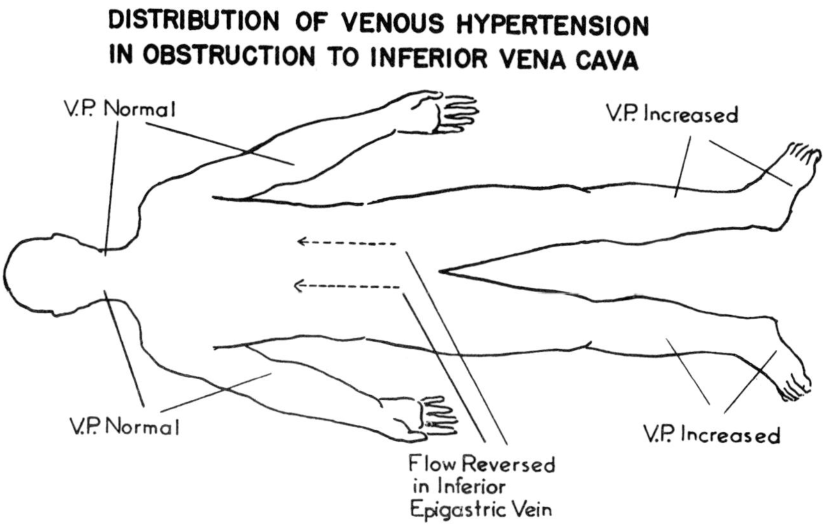

FIG. 138.—Obstruction to the inferior vena cava below the renal vein causes elevation in pressure in the veins of the legs and lower portions of the abdomen and reversal of venous blood flow in the inferior epigastric veins.

is reversed, *i. e.*, cephalad instead of caudad. The pressure in the tributaries of the superior vena cava, of course, remains normal. These differences must be ascertained in order to exclude generalized elevations in venous pressure and to localize the obstruction to the inferior vena cava.

Circumstances may exist in which the collateral circulation is highly developed, so that obstruction to the inferior vena cava may occur without elevation of the pressure within its tributaries beyond the normal maximum. This has been observed in several patients who had a therapeutic ligation and severance of the inferior vena cava below the renal vein.

If obstruction of the inferior vena cava is above the level of the renal veins, renal function will be greatly disturbed, the urine will be abnormal (oliguria, proteinuria, hematuria, and appearance of abnormal numbers and types of renal casts), and there will be venous hypertension limited to the tributaries of the inferior vena cava discussed previously.

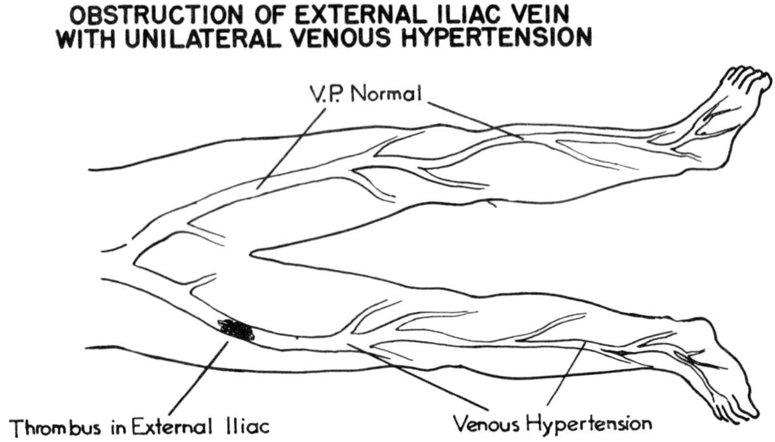

FIG. 139.—Obstruction of an external iliac vein. Venous hypertension is present in tributaries of the vein. The pressure in the veins of the other leg is normal.

b) *External Iliac Veins.*—Obstruction to the external iliac vein results in venous hypertension in its tributaries (Fig. 139). The additional observation of normal pressure in the homologous veins of the contralateral side indicates that the obstruction is localized to the one external iliac vein.

c) *External Jugular Vein.*—Obstruction to the external jugular vein results in venous hypertension in its tributaries located in the neck and

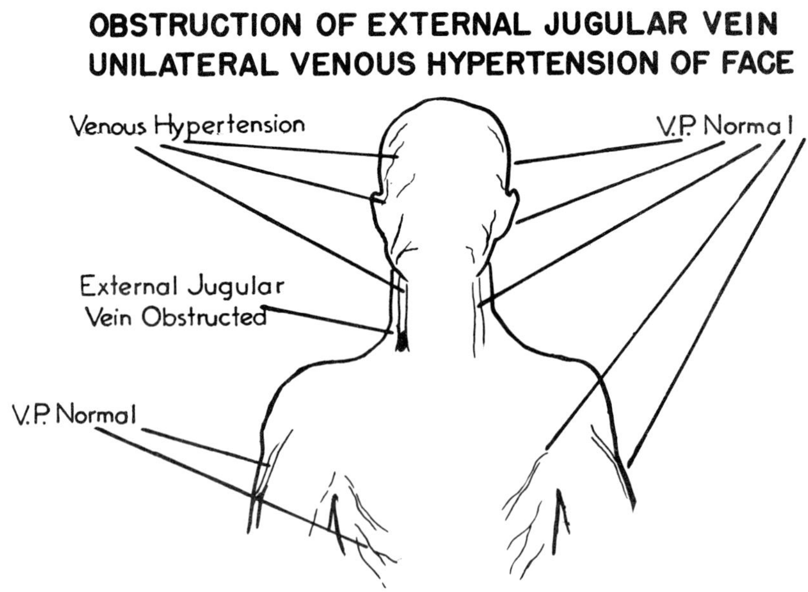

FIG. 140.—Obstruction to the external jugular vein. Venous hypertension is found only in its tributaries.

face (Fig. 140). The pressure in veins of the opposite side of the neck and face and of the arms and chest is normal.

d) *Portal Venous System.*—The pressure in the portal veins is increased in the presence of fibrotic disease of the liver as well as of other local diseases producing obstruction to the portal vein. In hepatic cirrhosis the portal vein and hepatic sinusoids are occluded to a variable degree by the contracting fibrous tissue, and portal venous hypertension ensues (Fig. 141).

PORTAL HYPERTENSION IN HEPATIC CIRRHOSIS

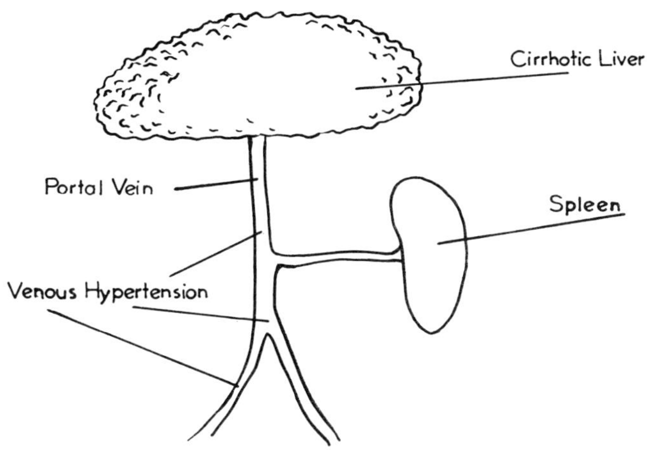

FIG. 141.—Cirrhosis of the liver produces portal hypertension.

In some instances in the collateral veins of the abdomen, such as the inferior epigastric veins, there is not only reversal of blood flow but venous hypertension as well. Unfortunately, considerable overlapping in levels of venous pressure in the inferior epigastric and other veins of the abdominal wall of the normal subject and of the patient with hepatic cirrhosis limits the accuracy of interpretation of any single measurement of venous pressure in the diagnosis of portal obstruction. It is also unfortunate that the pressure in the portal veins cannot be measured in the intact man. When hepatic cirrhosis is severe enough to cause caput medusae, a diagnosis of portal hypertension is easily established, and repeated measurements of venous pressure in the dilated veins of the abdominal wall render objective follow-up examinations more satisfactory.

Recent interest in surgical venous anastamosis to bypass the obstruction in portal hypertension of Banti's syndrome or hepatic cirrhosis focuses attention on determinations of venous pressure preceding and following the shunting procedure. The portal venous pressure in this disease varies considerably, usually exceeding 250 to 300 mm. of water. It may rise above 470 mm. of water but should decline toward the normal of 100 to 140 mm. after a shunting operation. Measurements of venous pressure should be made more frequently not only in the portal vein but also in all visceral veins during health and disease.

The principles concerned with the changes in venous pressure are essentially the same following obstruction to any vein. Edema and vascular disturbances may assist in localization of the obstruction. With adequate study and careful, exploratory use of pressure measurements, diagnosis and localization of the venous obstruction are easily established, and satisfactory therapy is facilitated.

Influence of Exercise on Venous Pressure in Venous Obstruction.—Muscular contraction in tissues drained by the tributaries of an obstructed vein produces a greater elevation in venous pressure in that network of veins than in the nonobstructed group on the contralateral side (Fig. 142). For

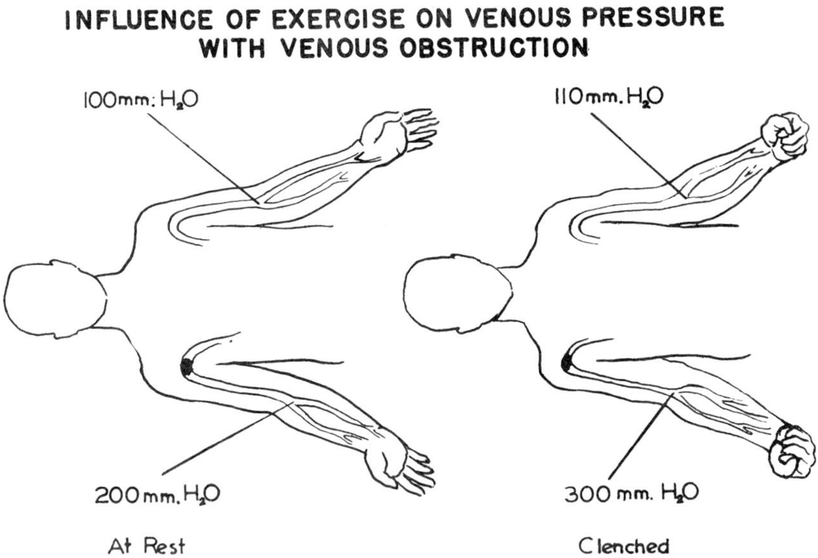

FIG. 142.—Tight clenching of the fists elevates the pressure in the median basilic vein in the presence of obstruction to the axillary vein. There is no such striking elevation in the normal arm.

example, when the axillary vein on one side is obstructed, clenching of the fist tightly several times will produce a much greater elevation in venous pressure in the median basilic vein on that side than will occur in the corresponding vein of the opposite arm with similar exercise. This is an extremely useful test which may be applied in many areas of the body when it is desired to substantiate venous obstruction. It is of particular value clinically in differentiating venous obstruction from lymphatic obstruction and in detecting slight obstruction. Until better standards for the influence of exercise on venous pressure become available, it is almost imperative to compare homologous venous networks on opposite sides of the body before any conclusions are drawn.

It is not sufficient to observe merely the degree of elevation in venous pressure following a standard exercise; the *rate of rise* during exercise as well as the *rate of fall* with cessation of exercise should also be noted. The more complete the venous obstruction and the less developed the collateral circulation, (1) the greater will be the rise in venous pressure, (2) the more rapid will be the elvation, and (3) the longer will be the time required for it to return to its original level.

The increase in venous pressure produced by contraction of the muscle is not only due to the influence of the pumping action of the muscular tissue pressure but is also probably due in part to the arteriolar and capillary dilatation associated with muscular contraction. This dilatation permits a greater velocity and greater volume flow of blood. Consequently there is a higher elevation in venous pressure as more blood is squeezed into the veins by the contracting muscles. This achieves venous distention, which is associated with extreme elevations in venous pressure for relatively little additional change in volume of blood squeezed into the veins by muscular contraction.

Etiology of Venous Obstruction.—Though measurements of venous pressure may be valuable in establishing and sharply localizing venous obstruction, they offer no assistance in determining the cause of the obstruction. This must be ascertained from *other clinical data.* Nor is the pattern of distribution of the venous hypertension helpful in this regard, since it may be the same for obstruction due to extrinsic or intrinsic neoplasia, contracting scars, phlebothrombosis, thrombophlebitis, or surgical ligation.

Degree of Venous Hypertension.—The degree of venous hypertension may vary considerably, depending primarily upon: (*a*) completeness of the obstruction and (*b*) degree of collateral circulation.

a) The more *complete the venous obstruction,* the greater will be the elevation in venous pressure. In general, the degree of venous hypertension *varies directly* with the extent of venous obstruction.

b) The more highly developed the collateral circulation, the less will be the elevation in venous pressure. In general, the degree of venous hypertension tends to *vary inversely* with the extent of development of the collateral circulation.

Determination of the degree of venous obstruction and state of development of the collateral circulation will become increasingly important with the development of new advances in vascular surgery which permit venous anastamoses to bypass obstruction and re-establish more adequate venous flow. This may be applied not only to the portal system but to almost all veins of the body, including those of the extremities.

CONGESTIVE HEART FAILURE

MECHANISMS

Because the rise in venous pressure in congestive heart failure is so consistent and because its variations are so closely related to the general state of the heart, measurements of venous pressure and their applications are of considerable assistance in the clinical management of congestive failure. Although the detailed aspects of the mechanism of congestive failure remain obscure, it is possible to appreciate the usefulness of these determinations with only general knowledge.

In chronic congestive heart failure the heart fails as a pump, that is, it is unable to supply the tissues with adequate blood to meet the needs under existing circumstances. For this reason and not because of damming of blood in the vascular system, the venous pressure rises. Venous pressure can rise only when more blood is "packed" into the veins (blood volume increases) or when the venous "tone" increases (the extent to which the veins squeeze upon the blood within them). It is possible that in congestive heart failure there is an increase not only in blood volume but also in venous tone. The chain of events occurring from the time of cardiac injury with subsequent insufficiency due to serious impairment of cardiac reserve and the development of increased blood volume and venous tone is not known. Regardless of this mechanism, however, venous pressure is conspicuously altered in congestive heart failure.

It is well at this time to review certain facts. Since, under physiologic conditions, blood is incompressible in the presence of sudden vasoconstriction, the volume of the vascular bed cannot change unless fluid escapes from the vessels, and this is not likely. Therefore, with vasoconstriction of the entire vascular system blood is forced into the veins where the pressure is lowest and the system is most distensible. Vasoconstriction is, therefore, not associated with a change in the total volume of the vascular system, except secondarily as a result of an increase in hydrostatic pressure, but merely with local changes in volume. When the blood volume is altered, there must be concordant alteration in volume of the entire vascular system but not necessarily a uniform one. The greatest change in volume will be in the venous system, for reasons previously discussed.

With chronic congestive heart failure the blood volume is increased, the veins become distended and venous pressure rises. The relationship of tissue pressure, edema and other factors to the venous hypertension is important but will not be discussed here.

Among the factors advanced today to explain the mechanism of chronic congestive heart failure are:

a) **Disproportion Between Cardiac Output and Rate of Venous Return of Blood** may produce a temporary and slight elevation of pressure in the systemic veins. The relative role, if any, of this change to the entire clinical syndrome is unknown. This alone, with the possible exception of pulmonary congestion in so-called "pure left ventricular failure," cannot produce the clinical syndrome of congestive failure.

b) **Increase in Blood Volume.**—Regardless of cause and effect relationship, it is generally agreed that there is increased blood volume in congestive failure and that it is responsible in part, at least, for the rise in venous pressure. It is also generally recognized that the kidneys do not excrete as much water and electrolytes during congestive heart failure as when the cardiac state is normal. This retention of water and electrolytes, with consequent formation of edema, is associated with an increase in blood volume and a rise in venous pressure.

c) **Increase in Tone of Veins.**—Some observers contend that the tone of the small veins is *increased* during congestive heart failure, so that the blood of the venous system is "squeezed" upon and the venous pressure is consequently elevated.

CHANGES IN VENOUS PRESSURE

a) **Right Ventricular Congestive Heart Failure.**—The concept of pure right or pure left ventricular congestive heart failure is most probably an erroneous one. There may be short periods of time or special circumstances in which there is failure of one ventricle or the other but in most instances both are simultaneously involved with the failure.

When the right ventricle fails to pump all the blood which reaches it from the great veins, blood will accumulate in the large, readily distensible veins without a notable rise in venous pressure. The left ventricle may then pump more blood than the right, but this will continue for only a few beats, after which time the output of the left ventricle would be determined by the volume output of the right ventricle. Both then eject equal volumes of blood, but the output is reduced and the tissues can receive less than the usual amounts of blood. This may be sufficient for the needs of tissue metabolism, in which case a new steady state in the circulatory circle is established with reduced output. On the other hand, if the output is not adequate for metabolic needs, neurogenic, chemical, renal and systemic factors become operative which *increase blood volume* by decreasing urinary output and incieasing the fluid compartments of the body. There may possibly be also an increase in venous tone or the tightness with which the walls of the veins fit around the blood therein. This latter may be part of a generalized increase in vascular tone or in venous tone alone. As a result of an increase in blood volume with or without an increase in venous tone, venous pressure is increased in the systemic veins (Fig. 143).

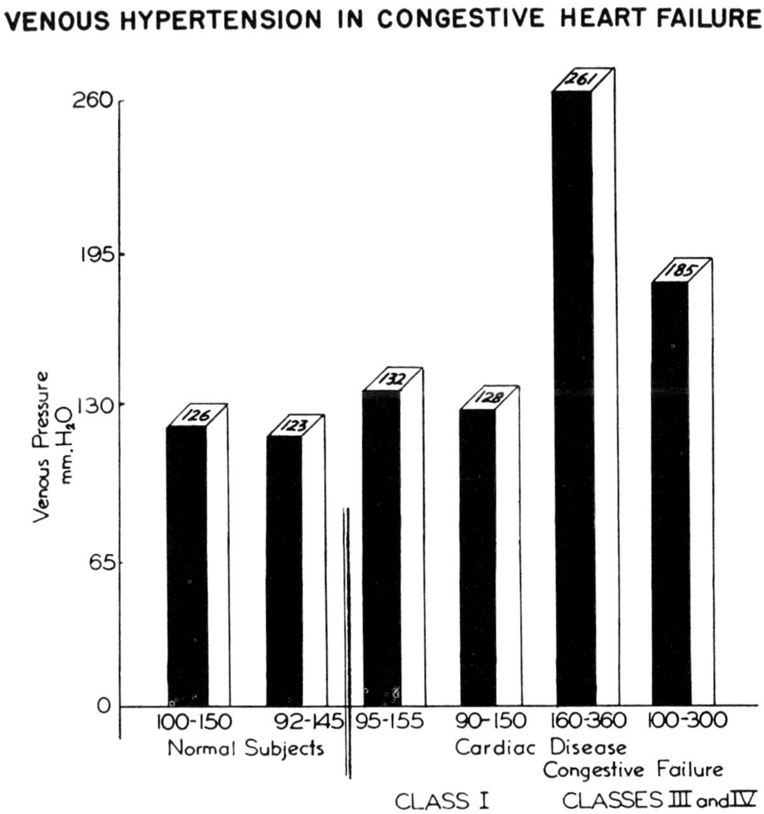

FIG. 143.—The pressure in the median basilic vein measured simultaneously in normal subjects and in patients with congestive heart failure. Values are indicated for functional Classes I, III, and IV. In each instance the column on the left represents the value with the subject in the supine position and that on the right with the subject in the sitting position.

The pressure in the median basilic vein has been observed to reach but seldom to exceed 400 mm. of water and ordinarily is recorded at about 200 or 250 mm. Except where indicated, the discussions of venous pressure in congestive heart failure will be limited to the systemic veins, since it is the pressure within these vessels that is observed in failure.

b) **Left Ventricular Congestive Heart Failure.**—When the left ventricle fails to pump onward the blood which reaches it by way of the pulmonary veins and left atrium, blood accumulates in the pulmonary system. If this continues for several beats, the pulmonary system of vessels will become congested, since its volume is relatively small and the volume of blood available to the right side of the heart in the systemic veins is relatively large. This accumulation of blood in the pulmonary system may produce dyspnea and pulmonary edema, and the clinician would say that "left ventricular failure" had occurred. The pressure in the systemic veins is not likely to change significantly because the volume of the systemic venous system narrows equally and simultaneously with loss of blood into the pulmonary portion of the circulation. If the venous tone is increased or decreased, there is a correspondent increase or decrease in venous pressure. Such a circulatory state may be satisfactory for the immediate metabolic needs and if the disturbance is mild, a new steady state is maintained with the alterations in distribution of blood volume and in pressure in the vascular system.

Apparently if this new steady state is not satisfactory, there are placed in operation neurogenic, chemical, renal and systemic factors which reduce urinary volume, alter the size of the fluid compartments of the body, increase blood volume, distending the systemic veins, possibly amplify venous tone, and elevate venous pressure in the systemic veins. Clinicians would conclude that "right ventricular congestive heart failure" had developed. It is evident from these discussions that the clinical and physiologic differentiation of pure right and pure left ventricular failure may be impossible except under special circumstances.

c) **Relative Values or Relative Venous Hypertension.**—Absolute or isolated values of venous pressure in congestive heart failure are often of limited significance, because the clinical syndrome may be highly developed with low or even normal levels in venous pressure. Of greater importance is the *time-course of venous pressure,* or the time-to-time variations, or the relationship of a given value to previously and subsequently determined values. For example, a subject may normally possess a venous pressure in the median basilic vein of 60 mm. of water, but this may rise to 120 mm. of water after the development of congestive failure (Fig. 144). The diagnosis of venous hypertension in this instance is based not on the higher level of 120 mm., which may be considered normal, but rather on the rise of 60 mm. above the measurement obtained before congestive failure appeared.

In most instances the level of venous pressure before the onset of congestive failure is not known and decisions must be based upon absolute values obtained when the patient is first seen. In doubtful cases a follow-up study after compensation will reveal the true significance of the initial values (Fig. 144), for the venous pressure usually returns to its true normal

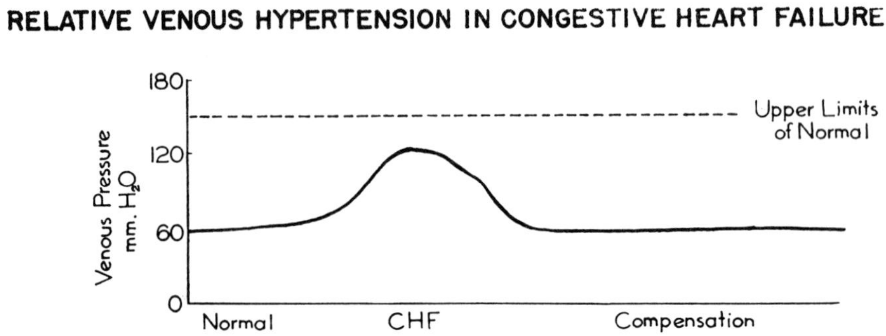

FIG. 144.—A definite elevation in venous pressure in a subject in whom congestive heart failure developed without the venous pressure having increased beyond the normal maximum.

level. A final decision is reached, therefore, in retrospect. With more extensive use of these measurements the significance of more precise evaluation of normal levels for each individual will be recognized and the interpretation of single and initial measurements obtained during illness will be improved. A graph of measurements before and during the course of the disease is therefore valuable, since relative venous hypertension may be as important as absolute hypertension.

d) **Influence of Phases and Course of Congestive Failure on Venous Pressure.**—Venous pressure varies considerably during the course of con-

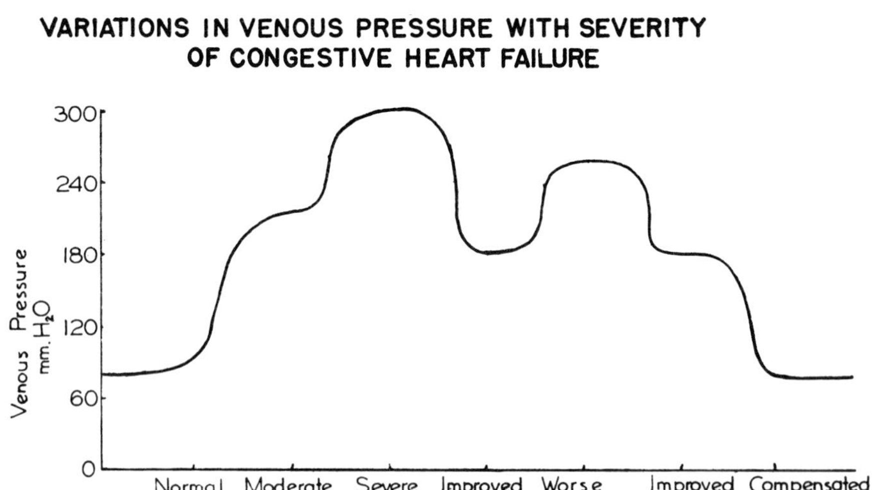

FIG. 145.—Variations in venous pressure with the severity of congestive heart failure.

gestive heart failure, elevations tending to vary directly with the severity of the disease (Fig. 145). As the failure improves, venous pressure declines towards normal, and with an increase in the degree of failure, it rises again. Once more a comparison of values is more elucidating than a single measurement. The error made by many clinicians of recording the venous pressure when the patient is first seen and never obtaining another measurement has been responsible for avoidable clinical difficulties.

e) **Lag in Appearance of Clinical Symptoms in Relation to Changes in Venous Pressure.**—The clinical symptoms and signs of edema, ascites, pleural effusion, hepatomegaly and cyanosis develop relatively slowly, whereas changes in venous pressure are more rapid and may therefore reflect a change in the cardiac state before many other aspects of the syndrome become manifest (Fig. 146). It is for this reason that such determinations are extremely important for charting the course of congestive failure.

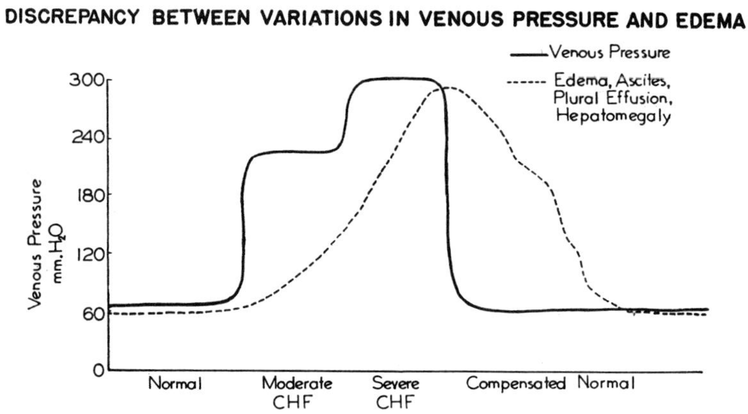

FIG. 146.—Graph showing the lag in development of many of the clinical symptoms in congestive heart failure. The venous pressure is a more sensitive index of the state and course of the failure.

The relationship of venous pressure to the edema and ascites of congestive failure is influenced by the pressure in the tissues. When the tissues are relatively firm, as in the youth, the venous pressure tends to follow directly the changes in edema or vice versa. Relatively little change in volume of interstitial fluid tends to be associated with a great change in venous pressure. In the senile subject, with loose flabby subcutaneous and other tissues, a large change in volume of interstitial fluid may occur with relatively slight change in venous pressure and vice versa. Cardiac compensation may occur in such patients with the venous pressure reduced to normal in the presence of a considerable amount of edema fluid in the loose tissues of the body. An apparent discrepancy between the degree of edema and the venous pressure is common in the senile subject and should be borne in mind in the management of these patients.

Because there is a considerable lag in the development and disappearance of the general clinical syndrome of congestive heart failure, measurements of venous pressure are often assumed to be unreliable as an index of the state of failure or as a sign of failure. This assumption, obviously, is not correct (Fig. 147). Venous pressure is one of the single most reliable and sensitive indices of congestive failure and of its progress. Interpretation of observations and correlation of various aspects of the clinical syndrome must, of course, be made in light of the lag between the development of the entire clinical picture and observed variations in venous pressure.

GENERALIZED VENOUS HYPERTENSION IN CONGESTIVE HEART FAILURE

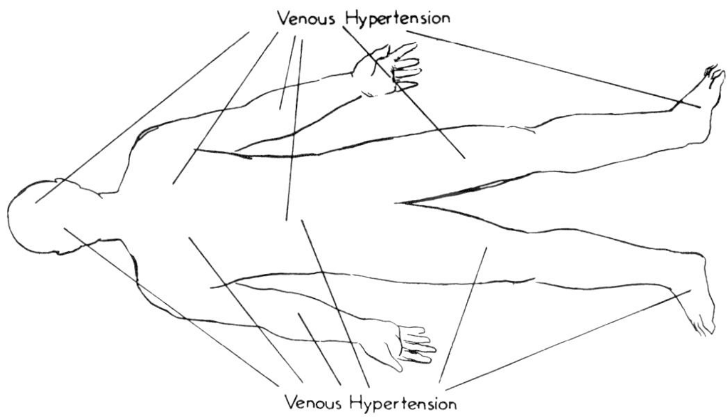

FIG. 147.—Venous pressure is proportionately elevated in all systemic veins in the presence of congestive heart failure.

f) **Generalized Venous Hypertension Due to Cardiac Disease.**—The rise in venous pressure observed in congestive heart failure is reflected in all veins; the pressure in the right atrium and that in the superior and inferior vena cavae is proportionately elevated. Therefore, all tributaries or all veins which finally empty into the inferior and superior vena cavae reveal an elevation in pressure. Obviously, then, the venous pressure in *all* systemic veins tends to increase proportionately in congestive heart failure (Fig. 147). This is an important diagnostic clinical manifestation provided, of course, the previously discussed phenomena are properly considered.

Several other clinical cardiac states that may produce generalized venous hypertension in the systemic veins are more appropriately discussed at this time, all of which are associated with an increase in blood volume and *vis a tergo* with or without an increase in venous tone if a great elevation in venous pressure ensues:

1) Cardiac tamponade
  a) *Pericardial effusion and exudation*
  b) *Hemorrhage into the pericardial sac.*
2) Concretio cordis
3) Persistence of the Network of Chiari
4) Tricuspid Stenosis

1) *Cardiac Tamponade.*—Whenever the pericardial sac is filled with any fluid (transudate, exudate, blood) under pressure, there results interference in the filling of the atria and ventricles during diastole (Fig. 148). This im-

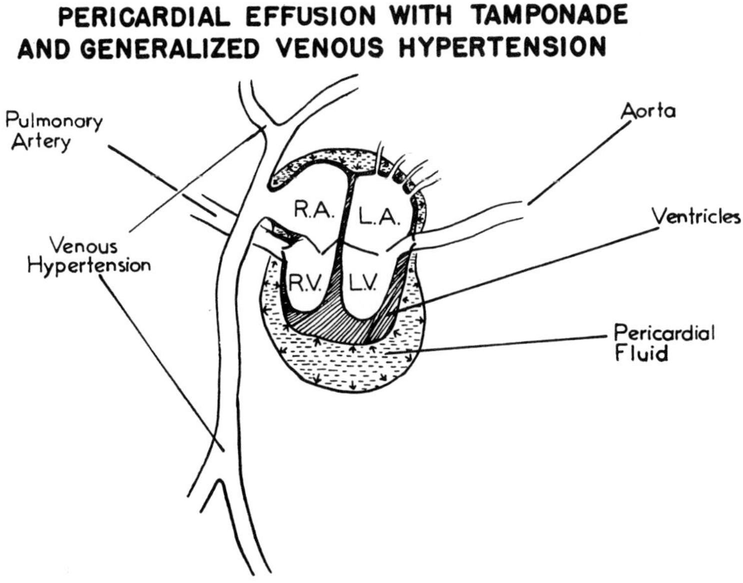

FIG. 148.—Fluid under pressure in the pericardial sac inhibits filling of the ventricles during diastole, increasing venous pressure in all systemic veins. Consult the text for details.

pairs the flow of blood through the right side of the heart, causes blood to accumulate in the superior and inferior vena cavae and in their tributaries, and effects an elevation of venous pressure symmetrically throughout the venous sytem. This type of venous hypertension may occur in association with pericarditis with effusion, a stab wound of the heart, or anasarca with the accumulation of fluid in the pericardial sac. The more rapid the accumulation, the greater the amount of fluid, and the higher the intrapericardial pressure, the greater the elevation in venous pressure.

When paracentesis pericardii is performed and the pressure within the pericardium is reduced, adequate ventricular filling occurs and the systemic venous pressure declines. Since the blood volume may increase during chronic tamponade, sudden release of intrapericardial pressure may not be accompanied by complete return of the venous pressure to normal. The previous normal level for the subject is attained when the blood volume again approximates the normal value.

2) *Concretio Cordis.*—Concretio cordis is associated with contraction of a fibrous coating around the heart (Fig. 149). This constricting encasement interferes with diastolic filling of the atria and ventricles and in turn with

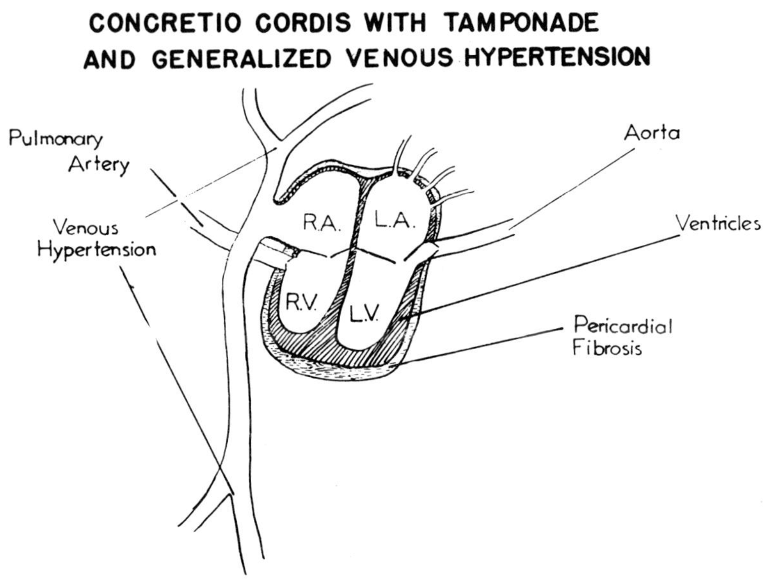

FIG. 149.—Cardiac tamponade is produced by concretio cordis. This causes a generalized and symmetric elevation in venous pressure in the systemic veins by interfering with diastolic distention and filling of the heart.

the flow of blood into the right side of the heart from the vena cavae. Increased blood volume with blood accumulating in the superior and inferior vena cavae and possibly an increase in venous tone causes the venous pressure to rise symmetrically within them and their tributaries in the same manner as described previously for pericardial effusion.

3) *Persistence of the Network of Chiari.*—In rare instances the network of Chiari persists as a congenital defect. These trabeculae stretch across the entrances of the superior and inferior vena cavae into the right atrium, obstructing the flow of blood into the right atrium (Fig. 150). A symmetric elevation in venous pressure throughout the superior and inferior vena cavae and their tributaries ensues.

PERSISTENCE OF NETWORK OF CHIARI WITH TAMPONADE AND GENERALIZED VENOUS HYPERTENSION

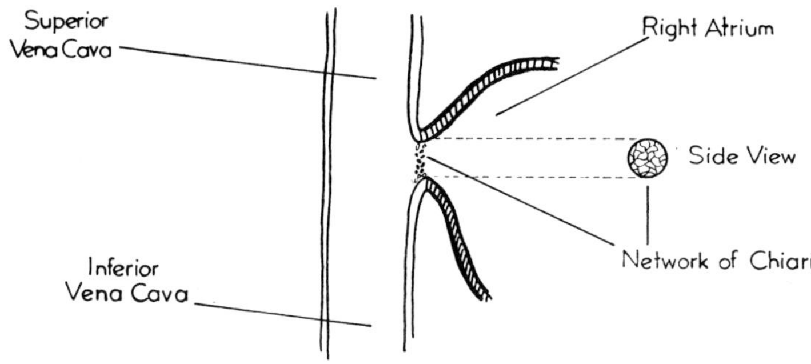

FIG. 150.—Diagrammatic views of the entrance of the superior and inferior vena cavae into the right atrium, showing the network of Chiari.

4) *Tricuspid stenosis* may also produce generalized and symmetric venous hypertension. This anomalous condition causes obstruction to the flow of blood into the right ventricle. The pressure in the right atrium is increased, as observed by cardiac catheterization, and the right atrium is enlarged. Some observers consider the elevation in venous pressure to be the result of congestive heart failure of the right atrium, and not simply a dam in the circulatory circle.

It is obvious, therefore, from the foregoing discussions that the degree of elevation in venous pressure in these four clinical states depends upon the degree of obstruction of venous blood flow to the right atrium or right ventricle. Venous pressure may reach levels as high as those in congestive heart failure or even higher. The limited number of studies of venous pressure in these states precludes the presentation of statistical data at this time.

Since congestive heart failure is the most common cause of generalized symmetric elevation in venous pressure, the differential diagnosis is usually not difficult.

HEPATOJUGULAR REFLUX

It has been known for many years that if there is insufficiency of the right ventricle, deep inspiration and pressure over the congested liver will cause engorgement of the veins of the neck or an elevation in systemic venous pressure. Hitzig described two methods for eliciting this phenomenon, referred to as the *hepatojugular reflux*, at the bedside:

1) The subject lies recumbent with his head turned slightly to make the superficial cervical veins more prominent. He breathes quietly and

regularly. While observing the jugular veins, the physician applies pressure (30 to 40 pounds of pressure) over the hepatic region with the palmar surfaces of both hands (Fig. 151). One of two conclusions may be reached:

a) If no visible change of the cervical veins occurs or if they collapse, then function of the right ventricle is *sufficient* at rest.

b) If a visible distention or increase in firmness to palpation of the cervical veins is observed, then there is cardiac *decompensation* or *insufficiency*.

TEST OF HEPATOJUGULAR REFLUX

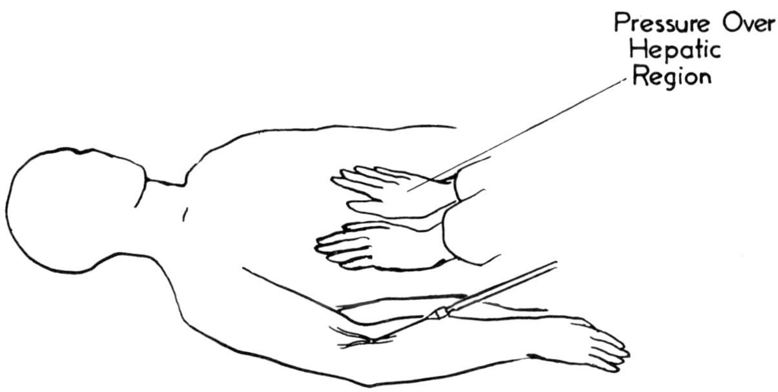

FIG. 151.—Method of applying the test of hepatojugular reflux.

This test aids in differential diagnosis, especially assisting in eliminating congestive heart failure as a cause for ascites, edema and hepatomegaly. Absence of the Pasteur-Rondot or hepatojugular reflux is almost pathognomonic of the absence of decompensation of the right ventricle. Exceptions will be discussed later.

2) The hepatojugular reflux test is made much *more dependable* when observed by means of measurements of venous pressure. Instead of merely observing the cervical veins, the physician determines the pressure within a median basilic vein with the subject relaxed and breathing quietly. After the venous pressure has been recorded with the subject relaxed and breathing normally, gradually increasing pressure is applied over the hepatic region for one minute. The maximum venous pressure during this procedure is then recorded. In about 90 per cent of normal subjects the venous pressure will decline 5 to 30 mm. of water and will fail to change in the other 10 per cent (Fig. 152). However in cardiac decompensation the degree of rise tends to vary directly with its stage. Venous pressure may rise to over 300 mm. of water with compression. Pressure over the lower part

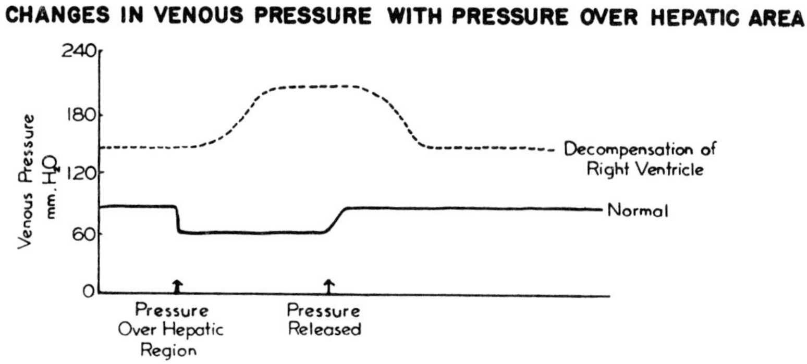

FIG. 152.—Variations in venous pressure with abdominal compression (hepatojugular reflux phenomenon) in a normal subject and in a patient with decompensation of the right ventricle.

of the abdomen will not produce dependable results in the hepatojugular reflux test.

Direct measurement of the venous pressure during the test is superior to the purely clinical procedure because it

a) is quantitative and permits comparisons,

b) is more accurate,

c) is more sensitive, and

d) permits observation of a decline in venous pressure, a phenomenon nonexistent in subjects with congestive heart failure.

Pressure over the liver and upper right part of the abdomen appears to produce its effect by squeezing blood into the inferior vena cava from the liver and abdominal viscera. Because with congestive failure there is an increase in blood volume, the veins are relatively full or distended and venous tone may be increased; the additional blood volume pressed out of the liver and splanchnic area into the more superficial veins of the body, as of the neck and arms, causes an elevation in venous pressure. Subjects with normal veins and normal blood volume have no difficulty accommodating the blood shifted from the liver and splanchnic area. Although the test is more sensitive with the subject supine, it may be applied with the subject sitting down as well. *The hepatojugular reflux test* is a sensitive test of early decompensation of the "right ventricle" and deserves more clinical use. When the results are negative, congestive heart failure is fairly dependably eliminated.

The hepatojugular reflux phenomenon may also be present in *cardiac tamponade* (pericardial effusion, hemorrhage, or concretio cordis). This may resemble, therefore, the reaction in congestive heart failure. Until the phenomenon has been observed in other disease states under different clinical conditions, final clinical evaluation must be deferred. It is, however, a valuable clinical test.

Exercise

The degree of elevation in venous pressure during exercise varies directly with the extent, vigor, and rapidity of muscular contractions. All things being equal, the rise is greater in patients with congestive heart failure than in normal subjects. This is due to increased venous tone, greater blood volume, and inability of the already distended veins to accommodate the additional volume of blood in the veins of the muscles available for muscular pumping, which is therefore squeezed into the already distended extramuscular systemic veins.

The influence of exercise on venous pressure in normal and diseased subjects has not been studied extensively. Certain experimental circumstances and contraction of groups of muscles have been investigated in man. Since the results of these studies apply only to special experimental conditions, they have no specific clinical applications and are, therefore, not discussed. For example, when a normal person rests in the supine position and alternately elevates and lowers each leg 10 times, the venous pressure in the

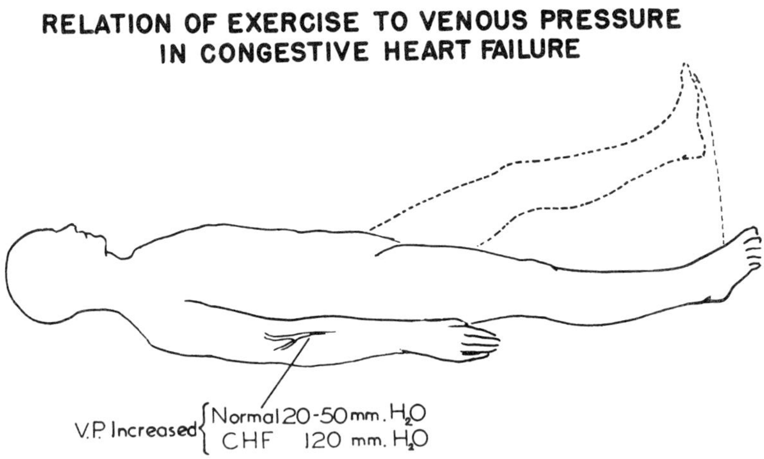

Fig. 153.—There is a greater elevation in venous pressure by a particular type of exercise in patients with congestive heart failure than in normal subjects.

median basilic vein rises 20 to 50 mm. of water, whereas patients with congestive heart failure experience an elevation of 120 mm. of water (Fig. 153). This, of course, does not indicate the change that might have occurred if the same subjects had been running, climbing stairs or a hill, or pushing a lawn mower.

DISTURBANCES IN CARDIAC MECHANISM

Acute disturbances in cardiac mechanism which interfere with cardiac output may increase the pressure in the systemic veins. The process is much the same as that described previously for congestive heart failure. The most common causes of reduction in cardiac output are paroxysmal auricular tachycardia, auricular fibrillation, auricular flutter, paroxysmal ventricular tachycardia and complete atrioventricular block. The chain of events which may follow are essentially the same as those described for congestive failure, *i. e.*, increase in blood volume and possibly increase in venous tone, producing the clinical syndrome of congestive heart failure with generalized and symmetric elevation in venous pressure. As stated previously, the increase in venous tone may be part of a generalized increase in vascular tone, or it may possibly be limited to the venous system, depending upon physiologic circumstances.

PULMONARY DISEASE

Disease of the lungs may impair venous return either by disturbing intrathoracic pressure or by obstructing veins directly. With a knowledge of the pathologic and physiologic processes associated with any pulmonary disease, it is possible to predict the changes in venous pressure. Although it is not possible to discuss each type of pulmonary disease, certain ones are presented to illustrate the manner in which underlying factors combine to disturb venous pressure and the manner of interpreting the changes clinically.

Elevation in Intrathoracic Pressure.—When the pleural cavity is filled with any fluid, the pressure within the thorax is increased in proportion to the amount of fluid accumulated. Not only is the absolute level of the intrathoracic pressure increased but also the degree of difference between the levels reached for the heights of inspiration and of expiration is reduced, the pumping action of respiration thereby being diminished. As indicated in Chapter 2, the normal negative intrathoracic pressure favors venous return to the heart, since it reduces the venous pressure in the great veins and right atrium and thus maintains the normal pressure gradient from the periphery to the heart or the "effective" venous pressure. Furthermore, the additional decline in venous pressure during inspiration produces intermittent reductions in pressure in the great veins and atrium. The resultant "pumping" action creates a pulsating flow. When there is fluid in the pleural cavity or cavities, the intrathoracic pressure is raised or the negative pressure may be completely eliminated. This reduces the pressure gradient (Fig. 154), and venous pressure rises.

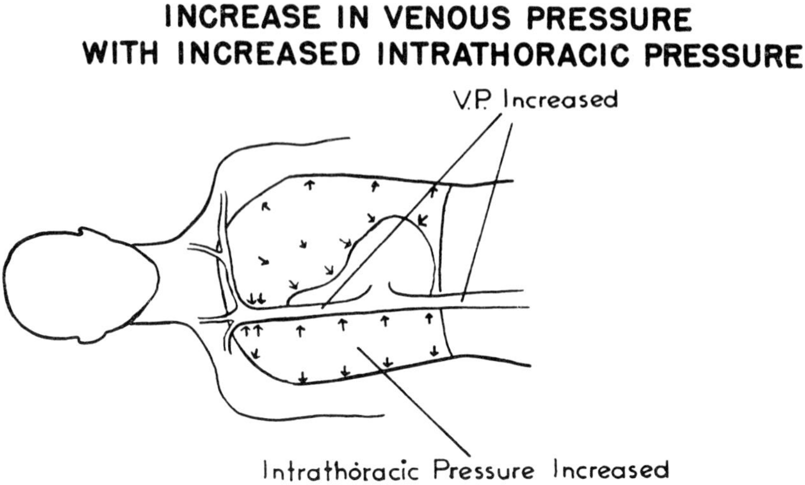

FIG. 154.—Increase in intrathoracic pressure impairs venous return into the thorax and elevates the pressure in the systemic veins.

In addition, the accumulated fluid in the pleural cavity interferes with the degree of pulmonary distention, excursions of the diaphragm and expansion of the chest. This in turn reduces the degree of fluctuations in intrathoracic pressure and the "pumping" action of respiration. Reduction in the efficacy of function of the thoracic pump retards venous flow and thereby elevates venous pressure.

Pressure in the systemic veins may rise only a few millimeters of water or it may reach levels noted in severe congestive heart failure. Because venous hypertension, dyspnea and other manifestations are also associated with congestive heart failure, difficulties in differential diagnosis between pulmonary disease and congestive heart failure may be encountered early at the bedside.

Venous hypertension may occur in pleural effusion, empyema, hemothorax, pneumothorax, emphysema, extensive pneumonia or in any pulmonary disease which increases intrathoracic pressure or interferes with respiration so as to impair expansion of the chest and the "pumping" action of respiration upon venous blood flow. It is important to determine the possible influence of disease of the thorax or lungs when measurements of venous pressure are made in the study of other diseases which may change the pressure within veins.

VARICOSE VEINS

Venous pressure in varicose veins has not received extensive study, but some important and interesting observations of practical clinical significance as well as of academic interest have been made. The more practical phases of these studies will be discussed.

1) **Effects of Increased Blood Volume.**—Because the veins of the lower extremities are dilated, their volume is increased (Fig. 155). This increase

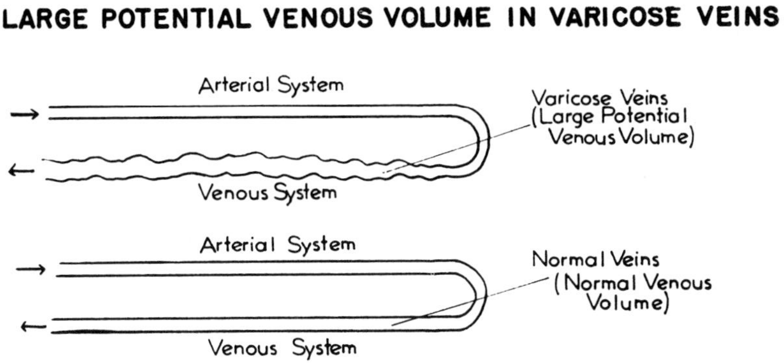

FIG. 155.—Varicosities increase the volume of the involved veins and, in turn, the volume of blood within them.

in space must be occupied by blood if the venous pressure is to be maintained, and the volume of the blood is, therefore, increased in proportion to the degree of dilatation of the veins. This may cause an increase in blood volume of 500 cc. With the diseased part dependent, the blood is held in the varicose veins but the extra volume of blood is "transfused"

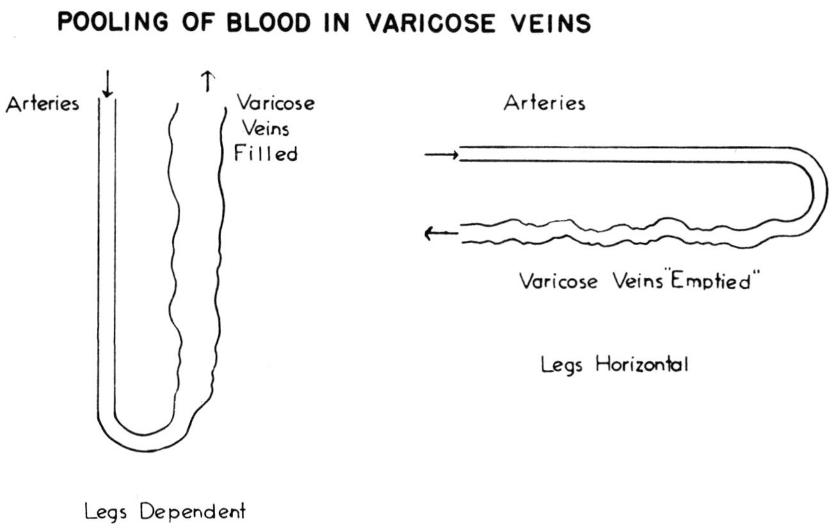

FIG. 156.—With the legs dependent, blood pools in the dilated varicose veins of the legs. This blood is rather suddenly returned to other portions of the circulatory system when the subject becomes supine.

or shared with other portions of the circulatory system when the subject assumes the supine position (Fig. 156). This "transfusion" increases the blood volume in the other veins of the body which are of normal volume and are in a normal physical state or tone; consequently the venous pressure rises several millimeters of water in the normal veins of the body.

2) **Local Variations in Venous Pressure.**—(*a*) *Effect of Gravity.*—With dilatation of the veins in varicosities, the valves become incompetent (Fig. 157). As shown previously (Chapter 1, page 31), when the subject stands,

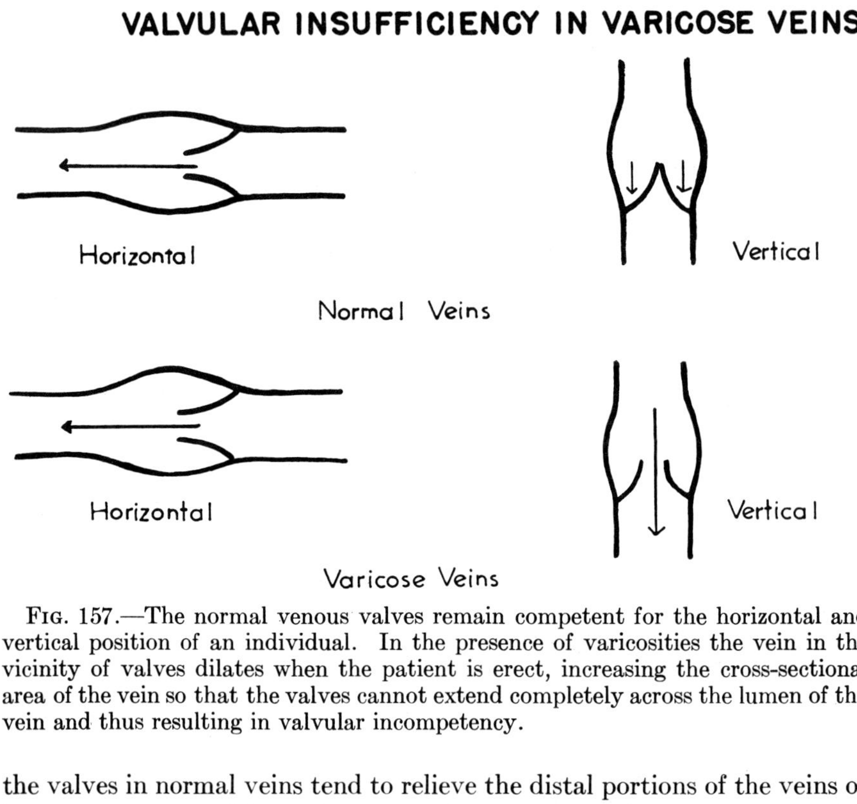

FIG. 157.—The normal venous valves remain competent for the horizontal and vertical position of an individual. In the presence of varicosities the vein in the vicinity of valves dilates when the patient is erect, increasing the cross-sectional area of the vein so that the valves cannot extend completely across the lumen of the vein and thus resulting in valvular incompetency.

the valves in normal veins tend to relieve the distal portions of the veins of large amounts of additional pressure due to gravitational forces. In the presence of varicosities, however, the associated valvular incompetency results in the full force of gravity being supported at all times when the limb is vertical.

b) *Effects of Muscular Contractions.*—Normal veins with competent valves permit the muscles to have a "pumping" action and to transmit their pressure effects and forces in the direction of the heart (Fig. 158). On the other hand, when the veins are dilated and the valves are incompetent, the force developed by the muscles is transmitted not only in the

REVERSAL OF BLOOD FLOW IN VARICOSE VEINS

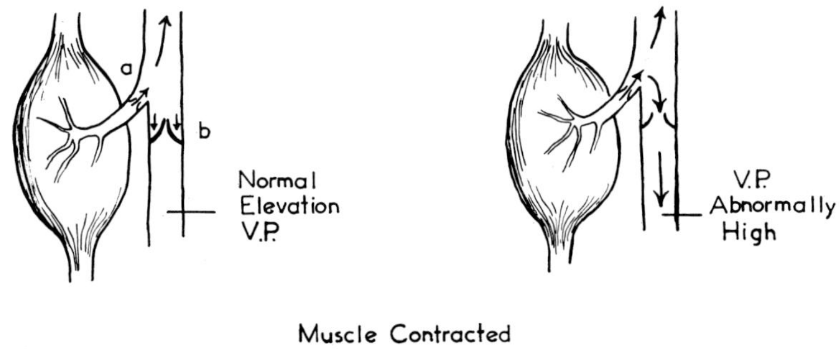

FIG. 158.—Diagram showing an incompetent valve in a varicose vein dilated in the vicinity of a venous valve. This increases the venous pressure in the veins below the incompetent valve and interferes with venous return to the heart during muscular contraction.

INCREASE IN VENOUS PRESSURE IN VARICOSE VEINS WITH EXERCISE

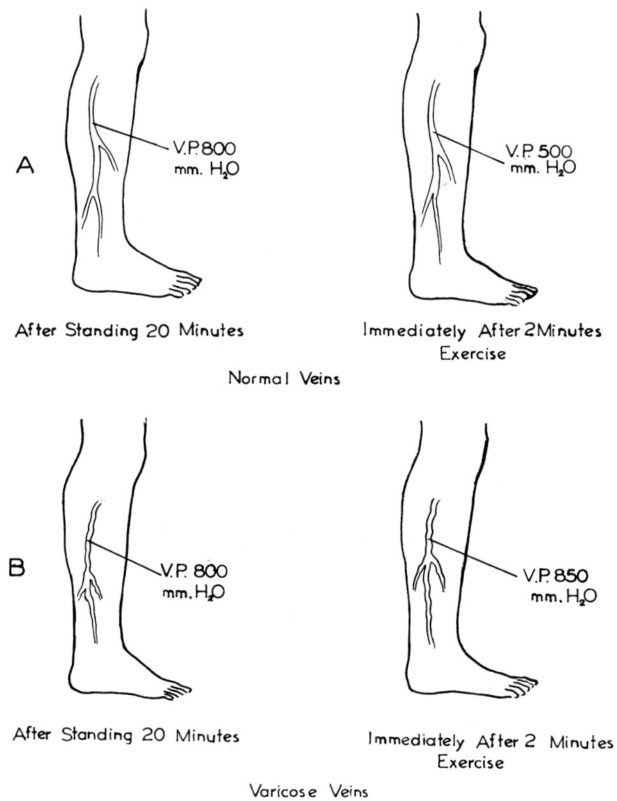

FIG. 159.—Exercise in the leg produces a decline in the venous pressure in the extremities of a standing man with normal veins, A, but an increase in a standing man with varicose veins, B.

direction of the heart but also away from it. This interferes with blood flow and may even effect a temporary reversal of flow in the legs. Valvular incompetency will cause a transmission of the pressure developed in the muscles to the veins in the lower part of the legs. Venous stasis ensues, with further distention of the veins and, in turn, more pronounced valvular incompetency. The hemodynamics in the veins is, therefore, progressively more and more disturbed and the pumping action of the muscles is impaired.

It has been suggested that measurement of venous pressure before and during exercise assists in determining the functional state of the venous valves. Normally, after a subject stands still for about twenty minutes and then exercises for a few minutes, there is a decline in pressure in the veins of the legs (Fig. 159). In the presence of varicose veins with valvular incompetency, exercise results in little change or even in elevation of pressure in the veins of the legs (Fig. 160).

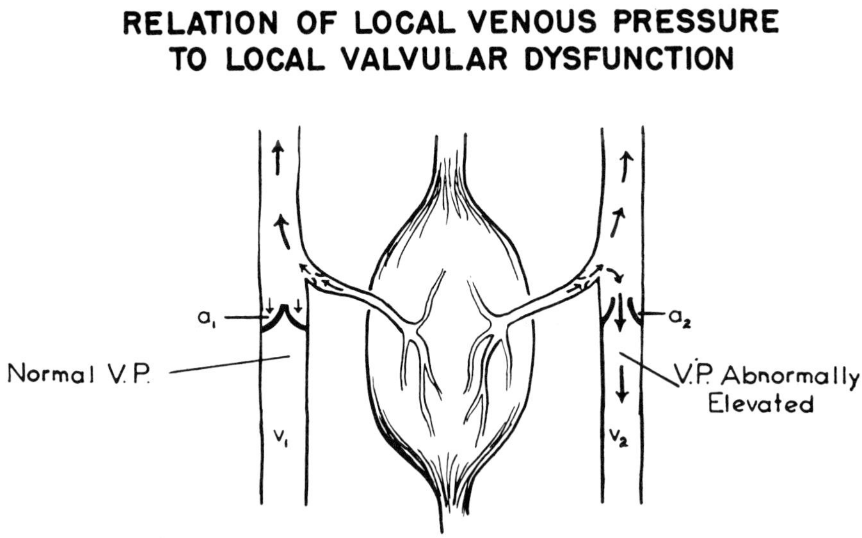

FIG. 160.—Because valve a_1 is competent and a_2 is insufficient, the venous pressure during contraction of the muscle is greater in V_2 than in V_1, both veins being located at the same level with respect to the heart.

Sharply localized dilatation in veins, due to incompetency of only one or two valves in a venous segment, will produce sharply localized differences in venous pressure. This is particularly true during muscular contractions (Fig. 160). It is necessary, therefore, in the consideration of such measurements in veins at the same level with respect to the heart, to realize that the differences in pressure may be attributable to valvular incompetency. Such differences are apt to occur in association with varicosities.

ARTERIOVENOUS ANEURYSM

Measurements of venous pressure in the vicinity of an arteriovenous fistula not only assist in establishing or confirming the diagnosis of the defect and in localizing it but also permit better appreciation of the disturbances in hemodynamics. When there is an arteriovenous fistula, either acquired or congenital, connecting the lumen of an artery with that of a vein, the high arterial pressure is transmitted to the vein (Fig. 161) and

EFFECT OF ARTERIOVENOUS ANEURYSM ON LOCAL VENOUS PRESSURE

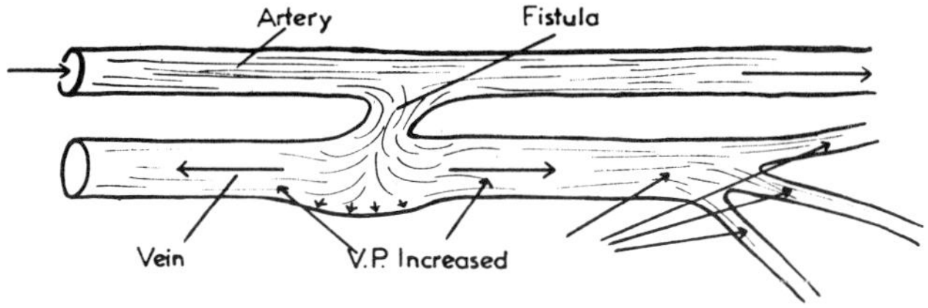

FIG. 161.—Arteriovenous aneurysm. The arterial blood under relatively high pressure flows into the vein, increasing the venous pressure.

produces local elevation in venous pressure within it and its tributaries. Venous hypertension occurs not only because the high arterial pressure is transmitted directly into the vein through a large opening but also because its effect is similar to that produced by partial venous obstruction from external pressure, such as a blood pressure cuff. In other words, the blood returning through the veins from the more distal parts must flow against the points of high venous pressure produced by the fistula. Competent and incompetent valves and variations in collateral circulation will influence the level of venous pressure in the more distal tributaries.

The pulsatile variations in arterial pressure with phases of the cardiac cycle cause the rate and volume of blood flow through the fistula to vary with the cardiac cycle, being greater during systole and less during diastole. As a rule, the flow through the opening is continuous, which accounts for the continuous murmur and thrill with systolic exacerbations in the immediate vicinity of the arteriovenous aneurysm.

Pulsations in Venous Pressure.—Obviously, the pressure pulsates in the veins directly concerned with an arteriovenous fistula, being higher during the systolic and lower during the diastolic phase of the pressure pulse wave. The closer the measurement of venous pressure is made to the arteriovenous opening, the greater are the pulsations in pressure, and the farther away, the less the pulsations (Fig. 162).

PULSATIONS IN VENOUS PRESSURE NEAR ARTERIOVENOUS ANEURYSM

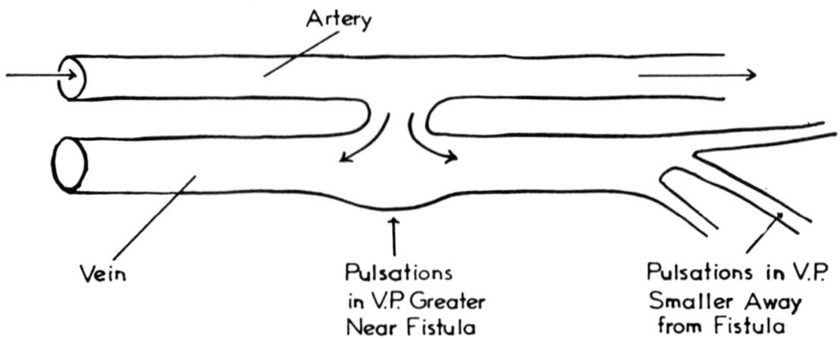

FIG. 162.—Pulsations in venous pressure highly developed in the vicinity of the fistula in arteriovenous aneurysm.

Degree of Venous Hypertension.—The magnitude of the hypertension in the vein and its tributaries varies directly with the caliber of the arteriovenous fistula (Fig. 163). Near the fistulous opening the venous pressure

EFFECT OF SIZE OF ARTERIOVENOUS FISTULA ON VENOUS HYPERTENSION

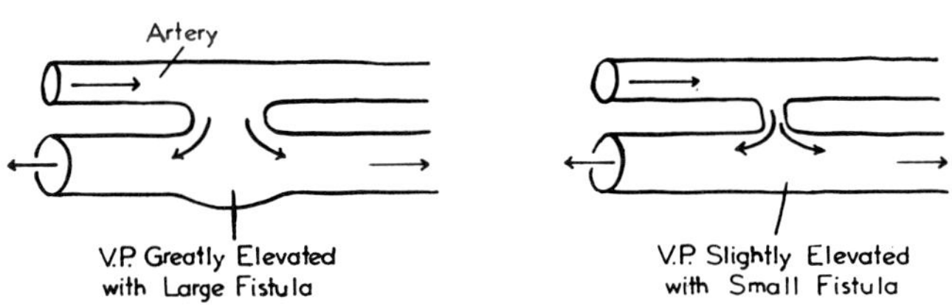

FIG. 163.—Influence of the size of the arteriovenous fistula on the degree of venous hypertension.

closely approximates the arterial blood pressure. The opening may be so small as to elevate the venous pressure only slightly. Because of the wide variations in the sizes of arteriovenous fistulae and in turn the considerable variations in venous hypertension, absolute values of variations in venous pressure observed by others has little significance when a given patient is under study in the clinic. As indicated previously for venous obstruction, comparisons in values obtained on the contralateral side have considerable significance in interpretation of the measurements. Pressures in involved veins may exceed 450 mm. of water, the elevation decreasing as the distance of the vein under study from the fistula becomes greater and the opening becomes smaller.

Localization of Venous Hypertension.—As stated previously, venous hypertension in arteriovenous aneurysms is found in the vein and its tributaries concerned with the fistula (Fig. 164). The corresponding veins

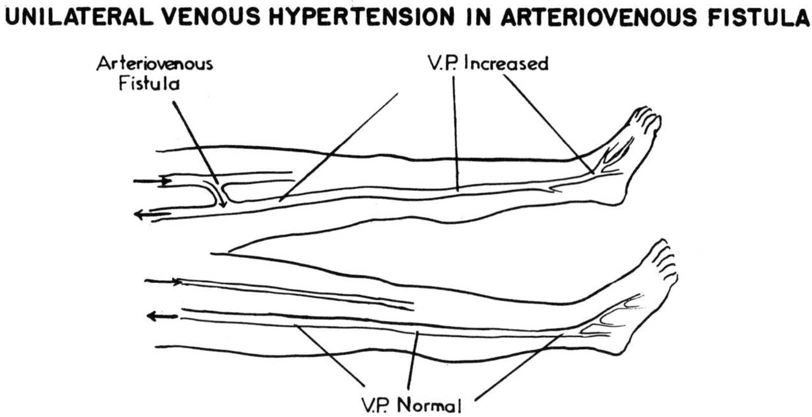

FIG. 164.—There is venous hypertension only in the involved vein and its tributaries in the presence of arteriovenous aneurysm.

of the noninvolved contralateral side exhibit normal venous pressure. This comparison in homologous veins is particularly useful in the presence of a small fistula, especially when the elevation of venous pressure on the involved side is within the upper limits of normal. By means of several measurements of venous pressure obtained in the veins involved in an arteriovenous aneurysm, it is possible to map out fairly sharply the location of an arteriovenous aneurysm, either acquired or congenital. The higher values and greater pulsations in venous pressure occur in the vicinity of the aneurysm. Other clinical studies must, of course, be applied in a patient as well, in order to establish the clinical diagnosis and to localize the arteriovenous aneurysm.

Effect of Closure of an Arteriovenous Fistula.—Closure of an arteriovenous fistula by surgical means or by external pressure applied locally over the communication causes a sharp decline in venous pressure in the involved veins, the degree of decline varying directly with the size of the opening. One may locate sharply an arteriovenous opening by means of observing the effects upon the venous pressure within the involved veins caused by intermittent opening and closing of the communication by means of external pressure applied over small areas (Fig. 165). When the exact location of an arteriovenous communication is not known or cannot be established with certainty, its localization may be determined in the following manner. After the pressure in a vein near the suspected area has been measured, with the venous pressure needle in place, pressure is applied firmly with the thumb over the suspected area until a point is found at which the venous pressure in the punctured vein declines sharply. The

REDUCTION IN VENOUS HYPERTENSION BY OCCLUSION OF FISTULA

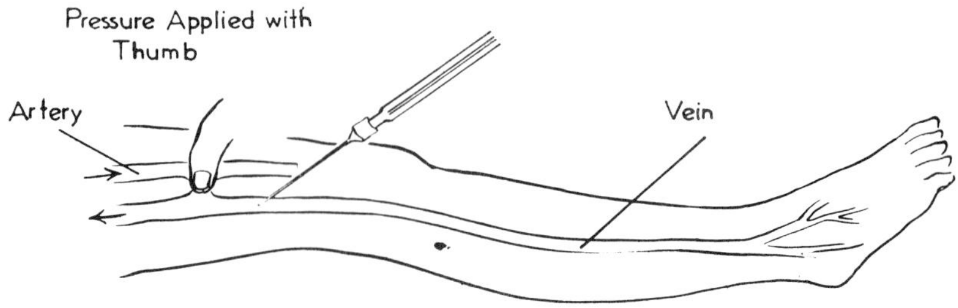

FIG. 165.—Pressure in the involved veins of an arteriovenous aneurysm declines towards normal levels when the communication is closed by external pressure.

fistula must exist underneath the area where external pressure produces a decline in venous pressure. Of course, many of the other hemodynamic phenomena besides venous pressure will be altered.

When the arteriovenous fistula is closed, disturbances in hemodynamic phenomena disappear completely, provided no permanent structural damage has occurred, and the venous pressure reverts to normal. However, if the veins are greatly dilated, valvular insufficiency is likely to be present, and varicosities, with the associated disturbances in venous pressure described, will be noted in the involved veins.

VENOUS SPASM

The influence of venous spasm on the pressure within the veins under study must receive consideration, for it may be responsible for errors in measurement. The spasm may be (1) local or (2) generalized.

1) *Local* venous spasm is common and is usually the result of the venipuncture incident to recording of the venous pressure (Fig. 166). The small needle employed with the phlebomanometer minimizes the incidence and severity of venous spasm. For accurate measurements the pressure should be recorded over a period of several minutes. If no change in venous pressure is observed, it is unlikely that local spasm is affecting the pressure recorded.

2) Venous hypertension may be induced by *generalized* venous spasm, as might occur from drugs administered immediately before a measurement of venous pressure has been obtained or simply from apprehension often associated with such a precedure. The elevation in venous pressure is due to a tendency to narrowing of the volume of the venous system (Fig. 167). The pressure within the veins rises as the walls tend to squeeze the blood within them. This type of venous hypertension, if not properly evaluated, may mislead the clinician in his interpretations of its cause.

INFLUENCE OF LOCAL VENOUS SPASM ON MEASUREMENTS OF VENOUS PRESSURE

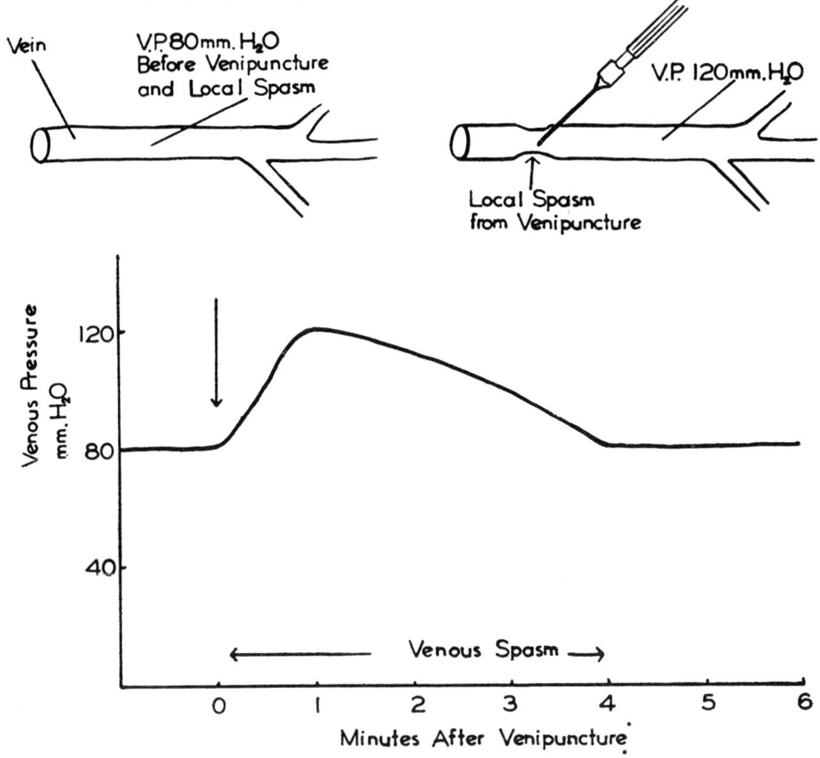

FIG. 166.—Influence on the venous pressure of local venous spasm due to the venipuncture. Graph shows the time-course of the venous pressure. The slow release of spasm with associated decline in venous pressure is illustrated.

GENERALIZED VENOUS SPASM AND VENOUS PRESSURE

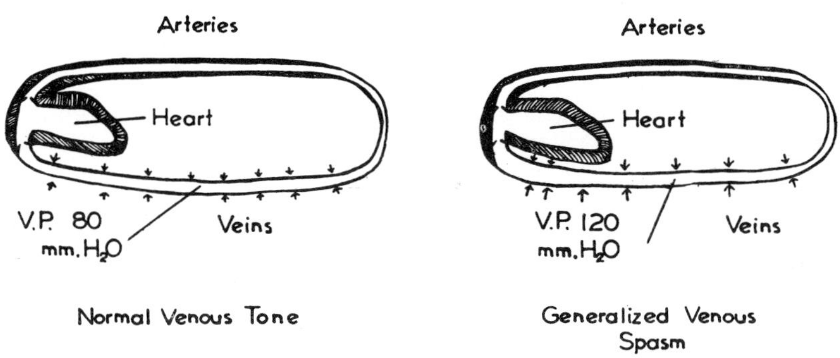

FIG. 167.—With generalized venous constriction the blood in the venous system is squeezed and the pressure within the veins is increased. Blood is shifted into the large veins near the heart, as indicated by a dilatation of the venous system near the heart in the diagram shown to the right.

SHOCK

The problem of venous pressure in shock is too complex and extensive to permit more than a brief discussion. In fact, it is not even possible to define the clinical state satisfactorily. Nevertheless, in peripheral circulatory collapse and shock, venous pressure may be profoundly reduced. The decline in venous pressure observed during a state of shock is either the result of a reduction in blood volume or venous tone or both. As stated previously, the veins are the main reservoirs of blood and possess the lowest pressure in the vascular circle during active circulation of blood. Therefore, any explanation of the venous hypotension in shock must be ultimately concerned with reduction in blood volume or reduction in venous tone (the tightness with which the veins envelop the blood within them) or in both. The disproportion between blood volume and tightness of the vascular system, the latter often referred to as vascular volume, is the important phenomenon. This *venous hypotension* may be produced by many factors:

1) **Reduction in Venous Tone.**—The tone of the venous system, like that in the arterial side of the circulation, may be reduced in shock and peripheral circulatory collapse. Relaxation in tone of the veins reduces the pressure within the veins (Fig. 168). Loss of venous tone is only part of the

DECREASE IN VENOUS PRESSURE WITH REDUCTION IN VENOUS TONE

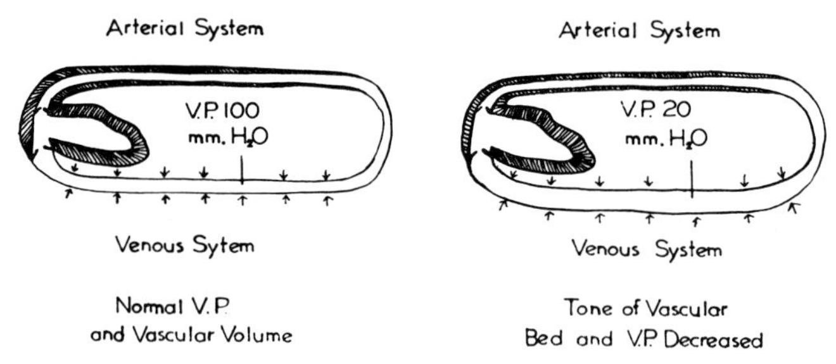

FIG. 168.—Reduction in tone of the veins with a decrease in venous pressure and a resultant increase in volume of the vascular bed.

hypotonus which occurs throughout the vascular system. Thus the walls of the blood vessels, including the veins, "squeeze" less upon the blood contained therein, and venous pressure declines. Blood may be distributed abnormally within the vascular circle and accumulate in the splanchnic and peripheral blood vessels. The abnormal distribution may be due not only to local differences in tone within the vascular circle but to other factors, such as hemoconcentration due to escape of fluid of the blood into the tissue spaces. Obviously, the volume of the vascular bed does not actually increase when vascular tone is reduced; this occurs only if blood volume also increases. In short, the decrease in vascular tone permits an easy increase in volume of the vascular bed, including the venous volume. Thus there is a potential increase in vascular volume.

2) **Decrease in Venopressor Mechanism.**—Not only is the venous tone reduced in shock but so is the tone of the muscles which assists in maintaining the tone of the venous system, at least the tightness of that part of the venous system which courses through the muscles. With a lowering of muscular tone, the veins dilate readily and their walls "squeeze" less tightly upon the blood contained by the muscles (Fig. 169). Venous pressure falls, the venous pressure gradient declines, eventuating in venous stasis accompanied by a reduction in venous return and a decline in cardiac output.

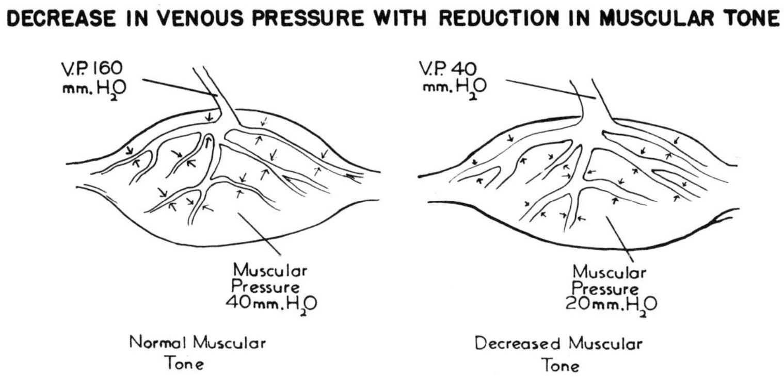

FIG. 169.—The pressure in the muscles "squeezes" upon the vessels coursing through them, thus assisting in maintaining pressure within them. In shock the muscular tone is decreased and therefore so is the pressure within the vessels, including the veins.

3) **Decrease in Cardiac Output and Vis a Tergo.**—With a diminution in cardiac output and arterial blood pressure, the *vis a tergo* concerned with the delivery of energy from the heart to the venous system and in turn, in part at least, with the maintenance of venous pressure, results in a decline in venous pressure and in venous blood flow. The extent to which the decrease in *vis a tergo* contributes to the venous hypotension in shock is unknown.

Other factors, such as disturbances in respiration and intrathoracic pressure, and hemoconcentration, resulting in greater blood viscosity, and greater friction with flow, encouraging greater transformation of kinetic and potential energies into heat, contribute to the venous hypotension in shock.

These same factors contribute in part and in various integrated ways to the venous hypotension observed in postural syncope, carotid sinus syncope, and syncope due to fright. For a detailed discussion of shock, peripheral circulatory collapse, and syncope the literature on these subjects may be consulted.

VENOUS HYPOTENSION

It is not possible to present the lower normal limits of venous pressure for any one vein in man or to indicate the hypotensive levels. It is difficult to establish definitely by a single measurement that venous hypotension exists in any one individual because of the wide variations in venous pressure in man. Venous hypotension is established with greater certainty when the previous measurements are available for comparison. For example, a

INFLUENCE OF BLOOD VOLUME ON VENOUS PRESSURE

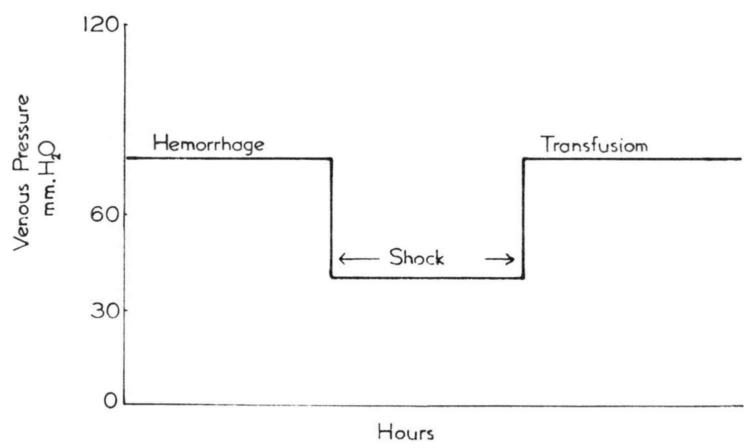

FIG. 170.—The influence of hemorrhage, shock and transfusion upon venous pressure.

venous pressure of 40 mm. of water in the median basilic vein may be found in normal man. However, if in a given person who had previously had a venous pressure of 100 mm. of water in his median basilic vein, peripheral circulatory collapse or shock is suspected and the venous pressure in the same median basilic vein under similar circumstances is found to be 40 mm. of water, then venous hypotension most likely exists.

Until more data have been accumulated on venous pressure, it will be necessary to depend primarily upon comparison of values rather than upon single measurements to determine the existence of venous hypotension.

Comparisons may even be made with values obtained after convalescence though this, unfortunately, requires interpretation in retrospect. For example, when blood volume is reduced by hemorrhage and shock occurs, venous pressure declines. With administration of blood, plasma or blood substitutes, the blood volume returns to normal, and the venous pressure increases to its previous normal levels (Fig. 170). As a rule, however, it is usually not difficult to correlate measurements of venous pressure with the clinical state during shock and following therapy.

DRUGS AND MISCELLANEOUS CLINICAL STATES

Venous pressure is influenced by many chemical agents. Drugs which produce vascular constriction, such as *epinephrine*, elevate the venous pressure, whereas those which dilate the vessels, such as sodium *nitrite*, lower the venous pressure. Intravenous fluids, especially colloidal fluids, affect venous pressure through their influence upon blood volume. Drugs do not influence venous pressure by virtue of direct action on the vein alone; their many other actions upon the cardiovascular system may contribute to the observed changes. It is therefore always advisable to consider properly the previous use of drugs or drug therapy during any interpretation of venous pressure.

The *digitalis* derivatives reduce venous pressure in congestive heart failure by improving cardiac function. The *xanthine drugs* may also lower venous pressure in congestive heart failure, probably by improving cardiac function, by direct effects on venous tone and by improving coronary blood flow, dilatation of the vascular bed, and reducing blood volume through their diuretic action. *Mercurial diuretics* reduce venous pressure in generalized edematous states, largely by reducing blood volume through diuresis. They may secondarily improve cardiac efficiency and the pumping action of the heart.

Venous pressure is elevated in *acute hemorrhagic nephritis*. The mechanism is considered by some observers to be due to associated congestive heart failure, to venospasm by some, and simply to an increase in blood volume by others. *Convulsions* are associated with rise in venous pressure because of the muscular contractions and the increase in intrathoracic pressure due to the Valsalva phenomenon and labored type of respiration during the convulsion. The pressure has been observed to rise 90 mm. of water, though variations are considerable. Anoxic disturbances in the autonomic nervous system and liberation of epinephrine contribute to the elevation in venous pressure through venospasm or increase in venous tone. The function of the entire venopressor mechanism is accentuated during convulsions.

GENERAL REMARKS

Although all diseases have not been considered nor has any clinical state been treated in detail, it is hoped that the discussions have indicated the significant role of venous pressure in clinical medicine. Satisfactory clinical medicine cannot be practiced today without proper consideration of venous pressure. Thinking in terms of hemodynamics within the venous system and of venous pressure will clarify many previously difficult clinical problems.

Standardization of methods and more extensive use of determinations of venous pressure will open new fields in medicine. Investigations involving the veins have been neglected and many problems concerned with venous pressure require further investigation in the clinic and laboratory. It is hoped that greater interest will be stimulated in the field and that clinical and laboratory investigations will increase to fill the gaps in the present state of knowledge.

INDEX

G

H

I